Older than a thousand lives,
It's deeper than a gene.
Beneath yet in the blood it thrives,
Where Spirit is the mean.

Contained within the mortal flesh,
This realm of brilliance waits.
To grow and spread its light afresh,
Through those who dare its gates.

EIGHTEEN BUDDHA HANDS QIGONG

By Larry Johnson, O.M.D., L.A.C.

Photography - David Schanaker
Model - Erika Trice Schanaker
Desktop Publishing/Design - Julie Van Leuvan
Cover Graphics - Darrell Perry
Cover Photography - Buddha Head by Jon Macker
Model by Jude Sullivan
Cover Model - Larry Johnson

Published by White Elephant Monastery

P.O. Box 261
Crestone, Colorado 81131 USA
http://www.virtualguild.com/elephant

Second Printing 1999
Printed in the USA on recycled paper
ISBN Number 0-924071-02-8

NOTE TO READER AND DISCLAIMER

Table of Contents

INTRODUCTION

Throughout history, peoples in many parts of the world have sought ways to develop their energetic potentials for improved health, martial power, and to bring themselves closer to the divine. In China these practices are called QiGong.

Man is a complex organism whose life is supported by countless metabolic changes. These changes are described as the interaction between Yin and Yang.

QiGong systems are composed of psycho pneumatic exercises that seek to balance these interactions through the regulation of the body, breath, and mind. It is believed that the correct regulation of body, breath, and mind will harmonize yin and yang, balance Qi and blood, clear the energy/information channels, increase vitality, improve resistance to disease, and transform pathological energy patterns thereby prolonging life and nourishing the spirit.

QiGong primarily trains the flow of Qi (vital energy) in the body. As Qi is the commander of blood, regulating the Qi will regulate the blood. Regulation of the body, breath, and mind utilize the complex energy systems of the body to vitalize the flow of Qi and blood.

QiGong can enhance other therapies, prevent reoccurrence of many disharmonies, shorten the duration of treatments for many illnesses, consolidate results of treatment by other modalities, involve patients in their own healing process and be used as a primary therapy.

QiGong has been practiced for at least 4000 years in China. It is believed that 18 Buddha Hands QiGong was developed by Bodhidharma, the originator of Zen Buddhism, in the 6th century AD. Bodhidharma traveled from India to the Shaolin Temple in China. He found the routine of the monks at the temple to have left them in such a weakened state that they could not successfully complete their Spiritual work. After meditating for 9 years he developed three sets of QiGong exercises to augment their Spiritual practices as well as to increase their physical vitality. 18 Buddha Hands is one of those sets of exercises.

Because 18 Buddha Hands drastically increases the circulation of vital energy, several styles of Chinese Martial Arts adapted the system to develop internal power and enhance physical health.

For the same reasons, healers and people on a variety of spiritual paths can make use of these exercises to augment their practices while others can use them to help prevent illness and increase vitality.

The original set had 18 exercises. The set presented here has 18 sections of from one to three exercises each with a standing meditation position at the end of each. These additions to the original were made by past masters to add depth and balance to the practice.

Following the axiom, "TO FIND STILLNESS IN MOVEMENT AND MOVEMENT IN STILLNESS", the current version offers both dynamic movements with co-ordinated breathing and static standing with quiet mind.

18 Buddha Hands QiGong affects many different levels in the human being. Suitable for beginners and advanced practitioners alike, it positively affects the physical form of the body as well as the energy channels, organ systems, Chakras, Essences, and Spiritual qualities. It particularly works on linking the three Tan Tiens (*see pg 28*) and opening the Eight Extraordinary Vessels (*see pgs 12-16*).

CHAPTER 1

BACKGROUND

QI

Qi is defined as vital energy-in the large sense the "stuff" underlying all manifestation in the universe. Qi inside the human body is both a carrier and a message. It transfers both energy and information. Qi emitted from a QiGong Master contains infrared radiation, particle streams, static electricity, etc.

There are two general classifications of Qi inside the body, Prenatal and Postnatal.

Prenatal Qi (Source Qi) refers to the vital energy given to the human at birth from both parents. It is the basic matter (Essence) and native force that support the body's tissues and organs. This Qi is directly related to Ming Men and the Eight Extraordinary Vessels of the body (*see pg 11*).

Postnatal Qi is a combination of Qi derived from the food we eat and the air we breath that sustains our vital functions. This Qi is directly related to the 12 primary meridian/organ systems of the body.

Together the Prenatal and Postnatal Qi form the True Qi of the body.
True Qi is the source of energy used in daily life.

QiGong was developed to balance, harmonize, and enhance the True Qi for health and longevity and to transform the True Qi for Spiritual Development. QiGong exercises can also directly impact Prenatal Qi, Postnatal Qi, Essence, and Spirit - that which directs our life activities and links us to the divine

YIN AND YANG

Yin and Yang are the two opposing, yet interdependent and complementary aspects of all existence. They can be used to describe the relationships between the qualities of all things. Imbalances in any one or more of the Yin/Yang aspects of our being results in illness. Yin/Yang balance on the other hand promotes wellness.

The basic properties of Yang are likened to fire and the basic properties of Yin are likened to water.

Yang qualities are hot, bright, rising, expanding, daytime, Spring, Summer, external, etc. In the human body Yang relates to the top, back, left side, and exterior. The bowels are considered Yang inside the body and Heaven is Yang outside the body.

Yin qualities are cold, dim, sinking, contracting, night-time, Fall, Winter, internal, etc. In the human body Yin relates to the bottom, front, right side, and interior. The viscera are considered Yin inside the body and Earth is Yin outside the body.

Because Yin and Yang are so closely connected and interdependent, any imbalance in one of them will soon affect the other. They are involved in a constantly changing energetic play called life. The play is staged within certain limits called balance. When these limits are breached by either Yin or Yang, there is sickness. Death, signifying the total divorce of the Yin/Yang relationship, is the end of the play.

THE TWELVE MAJOR ORGANS \ MERIDIANS

According to QiGong theory, the human body is nourished, protected and balanced by a complex network of Qi transporting channels. From each single cell to all the tissues and organs of the body, it is these channels which maintain and support the process of life. There are several classifications of these channels including Primary Meridians, Luo-connecting Channels, Divergent Channels, Extra-ordinary Channels, Sinen Channels, and Minute Channels. Each has its sphere of influence and function in maintaining the health of our body\mind complex.

A study of the channel system for the QiGong student is much like studying anatomy for the medical student. Such an in-depth study is far beyond the scope of this book . There are numerous publications on the market that can do justice to this subject (*see bibliography*).

For the purposes of this book we will confine ourselves to addressing the Twelve Primary Meridians and the Eight Extra-Ordinary Vessels.

When we look at an acupuncture chart, it is usually the Twelve Primary Meridians with their associated points that are depicted. The Twelve Meridians run vertically and bi-laterally on the body, each connecting with an organ (or function in the case of the Pericardium and Triple Heater) but influencing a much larger orb in the body than the area directly covered by the meridian.

Six meridians flow through the arms and six meridians flow through the legs. The Pericardium, Heart, and Lung Meridians are Yin and flow through the inner surface of the arm from chest to hand. The Triple Heater, Small Intestine, and Large Intestine Meridians are Yang and flow through the outer surface of the arm from hand to head. The Gall Bladder, Urinary Bladder, and Stomach are Yang Meridians that flow from the head down the body and along the outer surface of the leg to the feet while the Liver, Kidney, and Spleen are Yin Meridians that flow from the feet along the inner surface of the legs to the chest.

The Meridians are grouped into Yin\Yang pairs with the Yin Meridians being considered internal and the Yang Meridians being considered external.

The Meridians circulate vital energy and blood, warm and nourish the tissues, and link and support the various structural and functional aspects of the whole being while providing the route for internal man to communicate with the cosmos.

Each meridian has specific locations where the deeper energies of the body may be accessed from the outside. These locations are called acupuncture points. Each point acts on the body's energy in a specific manner. This is called the function of the point. The functions vary from point to point, and from point combination to point combination. In other words, the function of a point can be altered depending on which other points are being stimulated at the same time.

YANG ORGANS

The main functions of the Yang Organs are to receive and digest food, to absorb nutrients and to excrete waste material.

The Gall Bladder forms a Yin/Yang pair with the Liver. Its main functions are to store bile and secrete it into the Small Intestine to aid digestion. It is the only Yang organ that stores a pure liquid (bile).

The Stomach forms a Yin/Yang pair with the Spleen. Its main functions are to receive and decompose food, temporarily store it, and pass it to the Small Intestine for further digestion.

The Small Intestine forms a Yin/Yang pair with the Heart. Its main functions are to receive partially digested food from the Stomach, temporarily store it while assimilating nutrients, and pass the residue to the Large Intestine.

The Large Intestine is Yin/Yang paired with the Lung. Its main functions are to receive waste from the Small Intestine, absorb part of the liquid, turn the rest to feces, and transport the feces to the anus for excretion.

The Urinary Bladder is Yin/Yang paired with the Kidneys. Its main functions are to temporarily store urine and discharge it when the proper amount is in storage.

The Triple Burner is Yin/Yang paired with the Pericardium. Both are functions rather than physical organs. Although the Triple Burner is classified as a Yang organ, it is really the combination of the physiological activities of three areas of the body:

The Upper Burner is the chest area and generalizes the functions of the Lung and Heart in transporting blood and vital energy throughout the body.

The Middle Burner is the epigastric area and generalizes the functions of the Spleen and Stomach in digesting food and absorbing nutrients.

The Lower Burner is the hypogastric area and generalizes the functions of the Urinary Bladder and Kidneys in controlling water metabolism. It is also the residence of our Prenatal or Source Qi which is our inherited constitutional energy.

YIN ORGANS

The main functions of the Yin organs are to manufacture and store essential substances such as Qi, Essence, and body fluids.

The Liver is Yin/Yang paired with the Gall Bladder. Its main functions are to store blood, nourish the tendons, and maintain the smooth flow of Qi throughout the body.,

The Heart is Yin\Yang paired with the Small Intestine and is considered the overall ruler of the body, home of Shen (the controlling Spirit of the body\mind complex}. Its main functions are to control the blood vessels and house the mind.

The Spleen (including the Pancreas) is Yin/Yang paired with the Stomach. Its main functions are to govern digestion, absorption, and transmission of nutrients to the body, keep the blood in the vessels, hold the organs in place, and nourish the muscles. It is also involved in water metabolism.

The Lungs are Yin/Yang paired with the Large Intestine. The main functions of the Lungs are to control respiration, regulate the water passages and nourish the skin and hair. Regulating the water passages refers to the functions of turning part of the body fluid into sweat to be excreted through the pores in the skin, controlling the pores, and sending part of the body fluid down to the Kidney\Urinary Bladder complex.

The Kidney is Yin/Yang paired with the Urinary Bladder. Its main functions are to store essential substances. dominate reproduction, growth, and development, produce marrow, control bones and receive air from the Lungs.

The Pericardium is Yin/Yang related to the Triple Burner. Its main functions are to protect the Heart and to relay orders from the Heart to the rest of the body.

Lung Channel

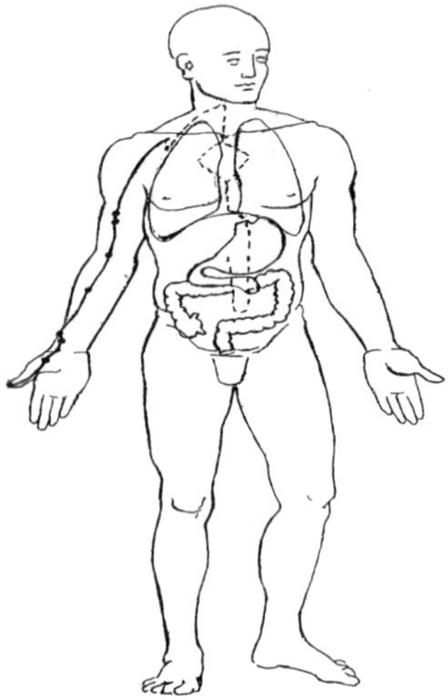

Large Intestine Channel

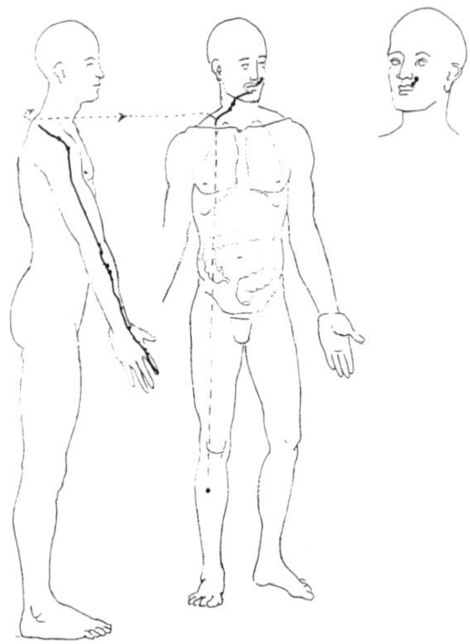

Stomach Channel

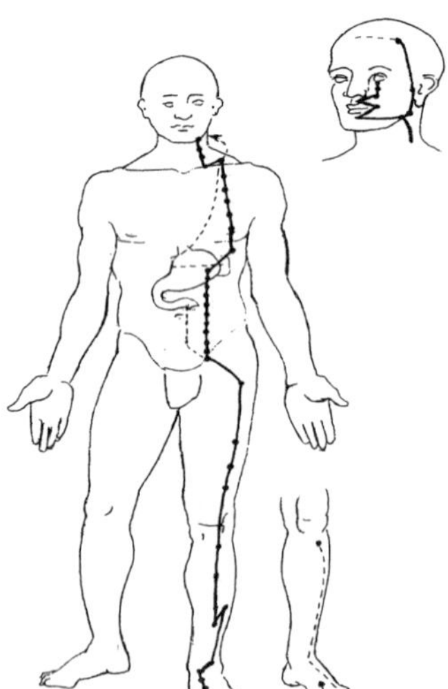

Spleen Channel

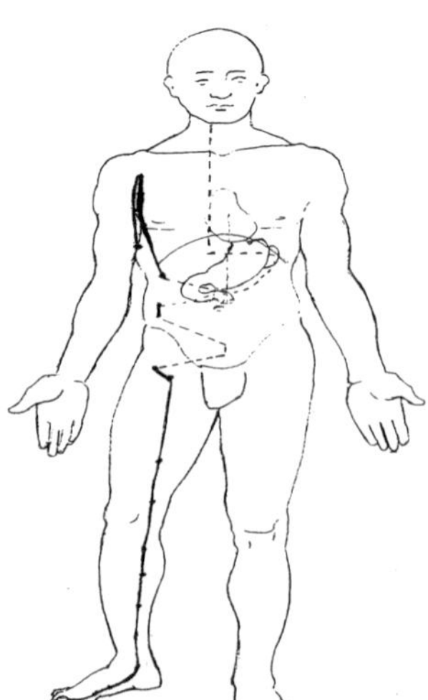

Heart Channel

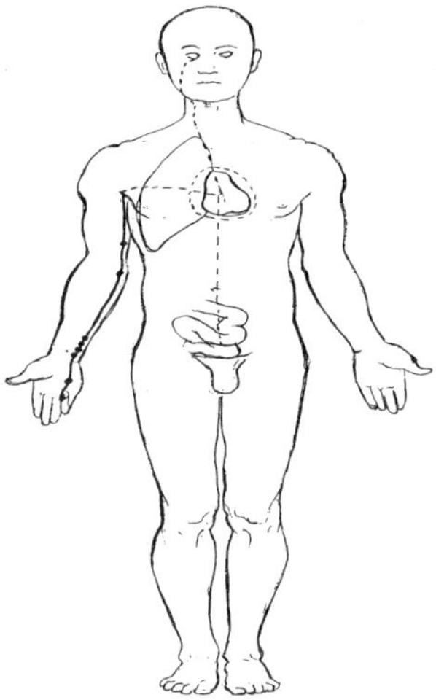

Small Intestine Channel

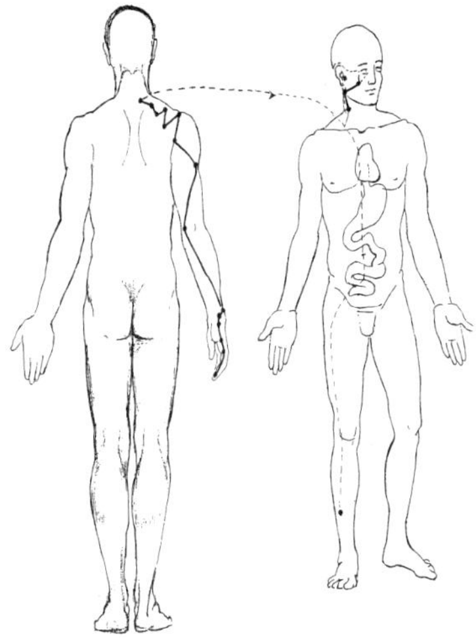

Urinary Bladder Channel

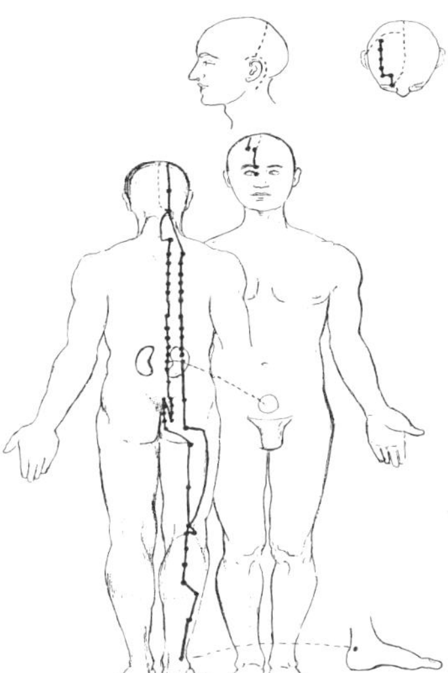

Kidney Channel

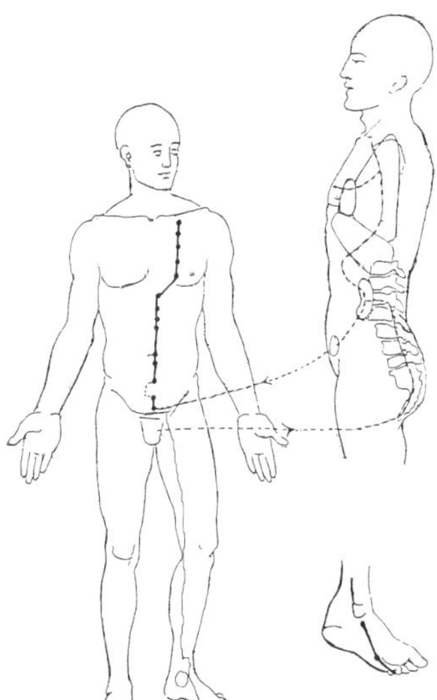

Pericardium Channel

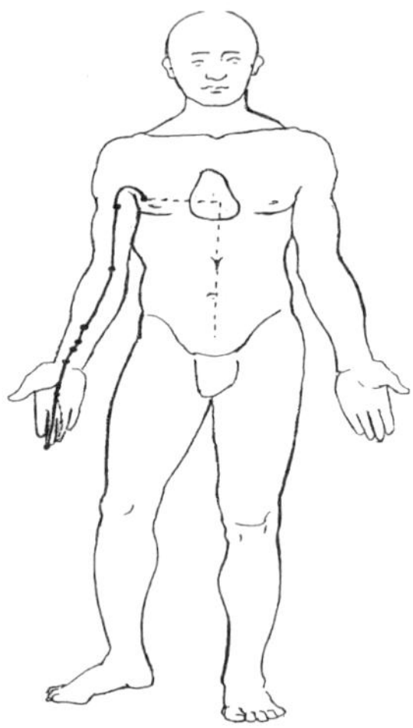

Triple Burner Channel

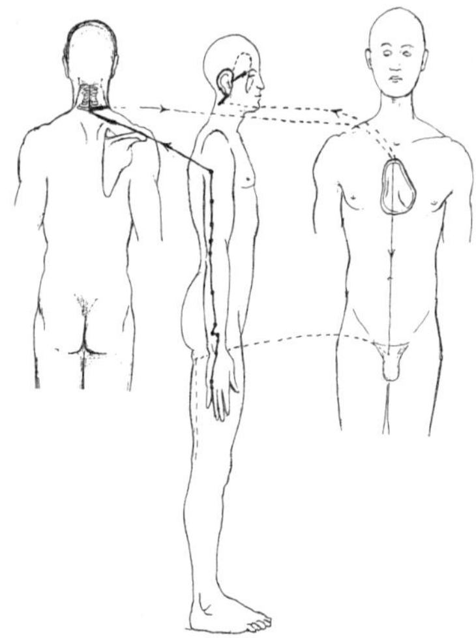

Gall Bladder Channel

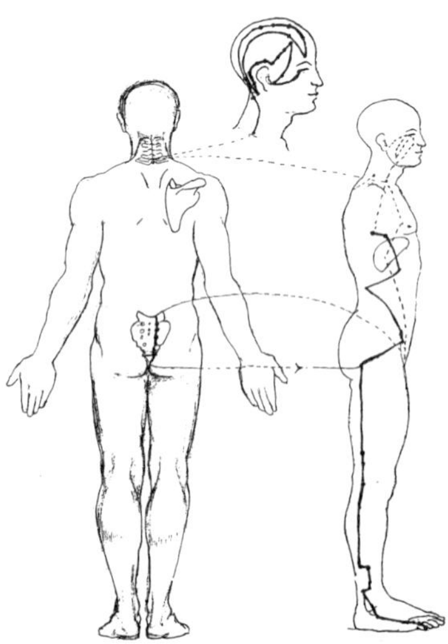

Liver Channel

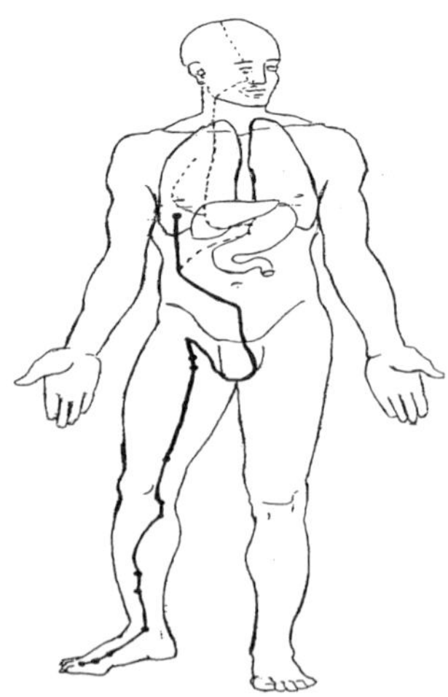

MING MEN

Ming Men is the first and most important energy center in the body. First because it is formed at the moment of conception before the fetus is formed and most important because it is the center of energetic transformations.

Bi-lateral Ming Men, located in the Kidneys, has seven energy channels connecting it's two sides called the Moving Qi between the Kidneys. Ming Men is where Heaven and Earth meet in man and interact to produce life.

Prenatal Qi, Postnatal Qi and cosmic energy interface and transform in Ming Men to support life. It is the origin of the Governing Vessel, the Conception Vessel, Chong Mai and the Triple Heater.

The Governing Vessel and the Conception Vessel are often considered the Yang and Yin branches of the Moving Qi between the Kidneys. Source Qi and Spirit are stored in the Ming Men.

Ming Men itself is often considered the back of the Lower Tan Tien. In fact, the Lower Tan Tien, Moving Qi between the Kidneys and Ming Men are so intimately connected that they can be considered one.

Ming Men

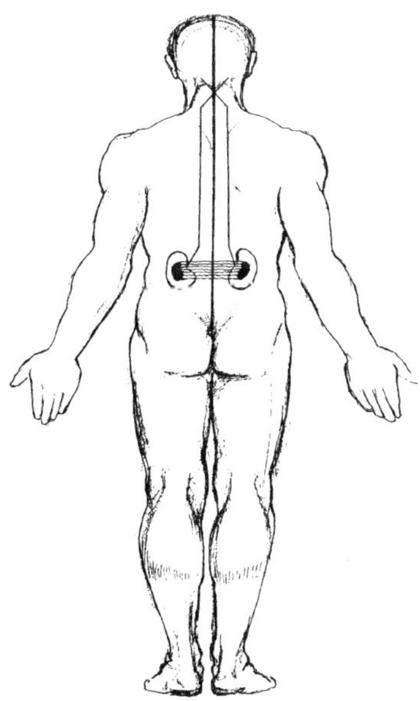

THE EIGHT EXTRA-ORDINARY VESSELS

The Eight Extra-Ordinary Vessels have a deep relationship with the inseparable structure\energy complex of the body and the exchange of information throughout the body.

At the first division of the fertilized egg the Governing and Conception Vessels are formed and at the second division the Belt Channel emerges. A child in the womb relies on the Eight Extra-Ordinary Vessels for all its body functions while the other channels of its body are being developed.

After birth, the Twelve Primary Meridians maintain life function while the Extra-Ordinary Vessels help regulate the Twelve Primary Meridians. The Extra-Ordinary Vessels act as reservoirs of Qi an Blood in the body, absorbing excess and repleting deficiency. They have direct relationships with the brain and spinal cord, hormonal control, the skeletal system, the genitalia, the circulatory system, the production of blood and the hepatic and biliary systems. Their influence on our body/mind/Spirit complex is deep and profound.

Each Extra-Ordinary Vessel has a Bi-Lateral Acupunture point (Master Point) that contols it.

DU MAI——GOVERNING VESSEL

The Governing Vessel, known as the Sea of Yang, helps regulate all the Yang of the body and through the acupuncture point GV 14 links all the Yang Channels. Du Mai controls the dorsal aspect of the body. The acupuncture point that controls Du Mai is Small Intestine 3.

REN MAI——CONCEPTION VESSEL

The Conception Vessel, known as the Sea of Yin, helps regulate all the yin in the body and links all the Yin channels. Ren Mai controls the ventral aspect of the body. The acupuncture point that controls Ren Mai is Lung 7.

CHONG MAI——VITALITY VESSEL

Chong Mai, known as the Sea of Blood and the Sea of the Twelve Meridians, is the main purveyor of Source Qi in the body. It strengthens the link between the Conception and Governing Vessels and is said to regulate the sinens and meridians of the whole body. The upper part of Chong Mo connects with all the Yang Meridians and the lower part connects with all the Yin meridians. The acupuncture point that controls Chong Mai is Spleen 4.

DAI MAI——BELT VESSEL

The Belt Channel circles the waist linking all the vertical channels on the abdomen. It has an especially close and binding relationship with the Conception Vessel, Chong Mo, Gall Bladder, Liver, Spleen and Kidney Meridians. The Belt Channel gets energy from the Liver and Gall Bladder Meridians and receives Source Qi from the Kidneys. The QiGong community recognizes its direct connection with Ming Men although this is not mentioned often in the Chinese Medical community. By regulating the vertical channels on the abdomen, the Belt Channel harmonizes energy

between the upper and lower parts of the body. The acupuncture point that controls Dai Mai is Gall Bladder 41.

YANG CHIAO MAI——YANG HEEL VESSEL

The Yang Heel Channel links the Urinary Bladder, Gall Bladder, Small Intestine, Large Intestine, and Stomach Channels. It is somewhat regarded as a branch of the Urinary Bladder Meridian. The Yang Heel Channel controls the amount and movement of Yang energy in the body, dominates activity and corresponds to the energy of Heaven. The acupuncture point that controls Yang Chiao Mai is Urinary Bladder 62.

YIN CHIAO MAI——YIN HEEL VESSEL

The Yin Heel Channel links the Kidney and Urinary Bladder Channels and is somewhat regarded as a secondary branch of the Kidney Meridian. It controls the amount of and movement of Yin in the body, dominates quietness, and corresponds to the energy of Earth. The acupuncture point that controls Yin Chiao Mai is Kidney 6.

YIN WEI MAI——YIN LINKING VESSEL

The Yin Linking Channel dominates the interior of the body, with an especially powerful effect on the Conception Vessel, Heart and Lung. It also connects with the Kidney Spleen, and Liver. Like the Chong Mai it contains Source Qi. It is mainly concerned with regulating the deep energies of the body. The acupuncture point that controls the Yin Wei Mai is Pericardium 6.

YANG WEI MAI——YANG LINKING VESSEL

The Yang Linking Channel dominates the exterior of the body, connecting with the Triple Heater, Gall Bladder, Urinary Bladder, Small Intestine, Stomach, and Governing Vessel. It is mainly concerned with regulating the defensive energy of the body. The acupuncture point that controls Yang Wei Mai is Triple Heater 5.

Each Extra-Ordinary Vessel has a bilateral Master Point (as mentioned above) on one of the limbs that activates it. The Vessels have their own functions and can be used therapeutically alone, but they have been shown to work very effectively in specific pairs. The paired Vessels support and augment the functions of each other. Dai Mai works with Yang Wei Mai—Du Mai works with Yang Chaio Mai—Chong Mai works with Yin Wei Mai—Ren Mai works with Yin Chaio Mai. The Master Point of one of each pair is on the upper limb and the Master Point of the other member of the pair is on the lower limb.

THE EIGHT EXTRAORDINARY VESSELS ARE THE PATHWAYS OF SPIRITUAL TRANSFORMATION

Governing Vessel - DU MAI

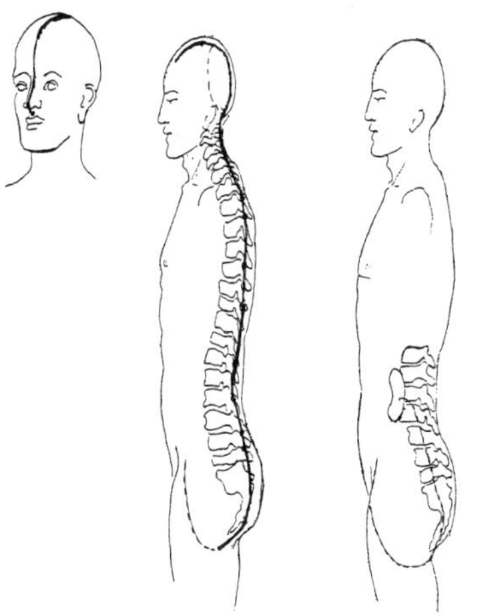

Conception Vessel - REN MAI

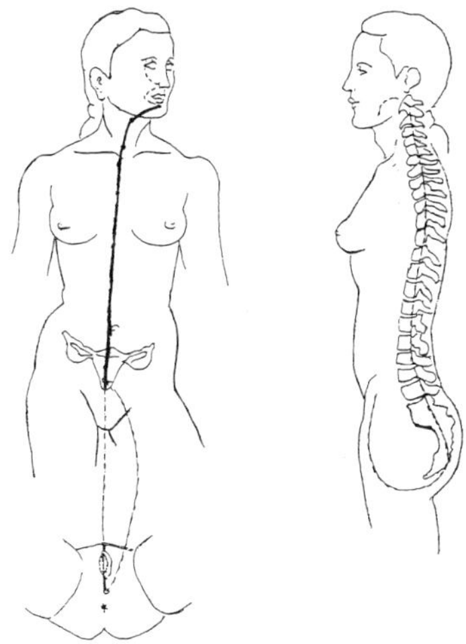

Vitality Vessel -CHONG MAI

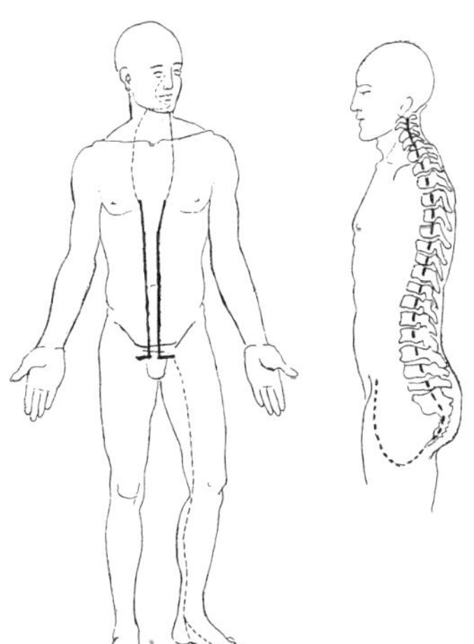

Belt Vessel - DAI MAI

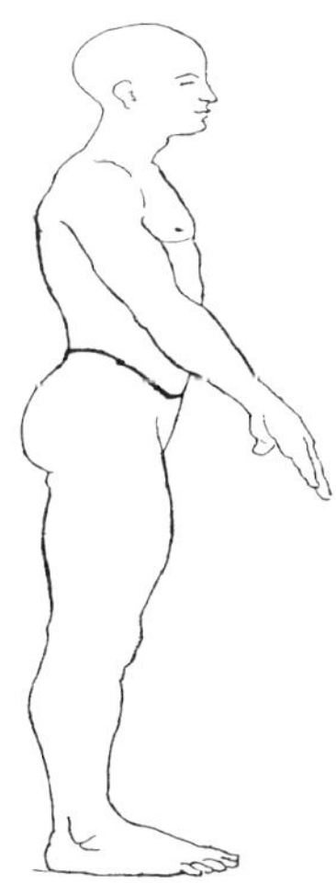

Yang Heel Vessel - YANG CHAIO MAI

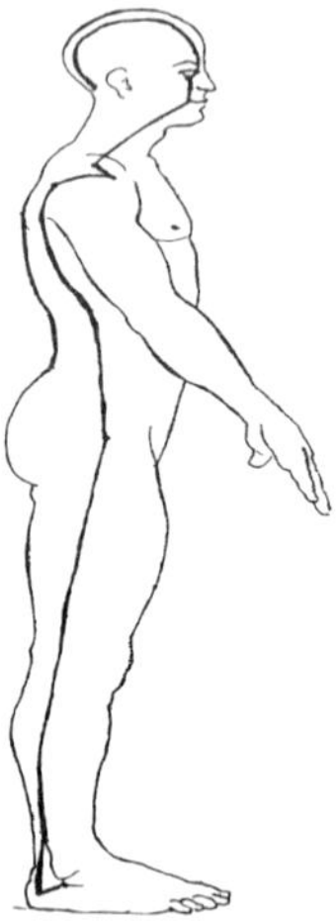

Yin Heel Vessel - YIN CHAIO MAI

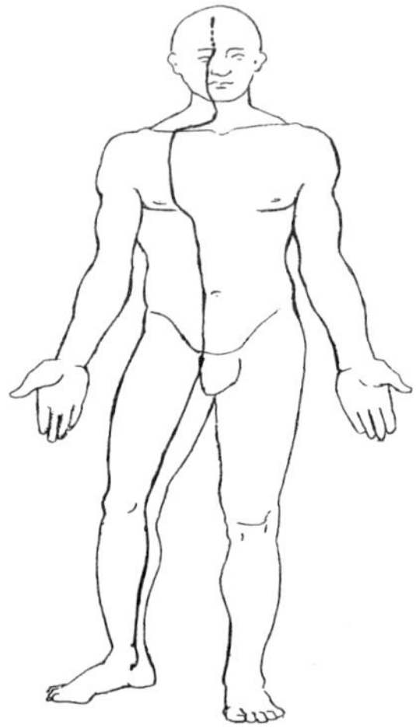

Yang Linking Vessel - YANG WEI MAI

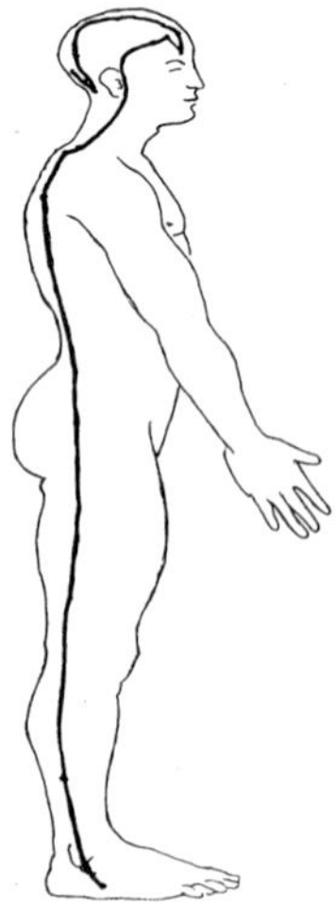

Yin Linking Vessel - YIN WEI MAI

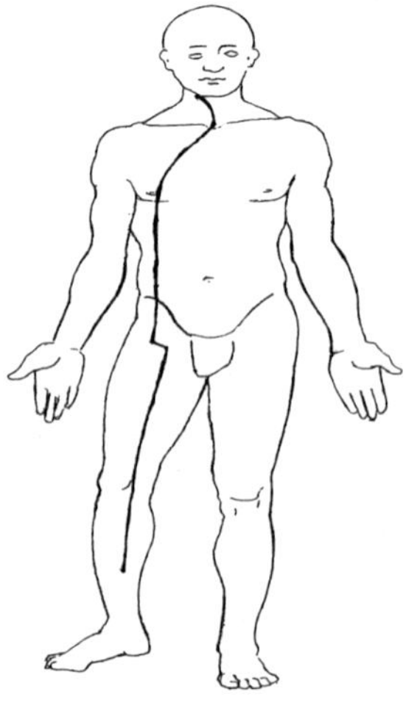

CHAPTER 2

QIGONG

QIGONG requires that the practitioner regulate the body, breath and mind. Body position is the base, breath is the activator and mind is the guide.

There are two basic types of QiGong—quiet and moving.

Quiet or static QiGong can be performed while standing, sitting or lying as long as there is no body movement. The emphasis in this type is usually on the internal organs and energy systems and utilizes the body shape and mind to move the Qi. The goal here is movement in stillness. The cerebral cortex remains relatively still in Quiet QiGong. Some Quiet QiGong positions are quite strenuous and also exercise the muscles, tendons and bones.

Moving or Dynamic QiGong requires movement of the trunk or limbs. This causes more excitement of the cerebral cortex. The goal here is to be externally active but internally still. Body shape, motion and the mind are used to move the Qi. In Moving QiGong, the internal energy systems and organs are developed as well as the muscles, tendons and bones .

THE THREE REGULATIONS

1. REGULATING BREATH

Breath regulation requires the control of the quantity, quality, duration and destination of the breath. Generally speaking QiGong requires your breathing to be of long duration on both the inhale and the exhale. A much larger amount of air is inhaled and exhaled than usual and the breath is qualitatively very soft. The destination is dependent on the specific exercise being performed. In some exercises these parameters change for specific reasons.

Breath regulation increases the efficiency of the oxygen/carbon dioxide exchange. This ensures the whole body and especially the brain has an abundant supply of oxygen and that waste materials are removed expediently. This in itself constitutes an inner cleansing process. Many of the positive effects of QiGong are directly related to this extra replenishment of oxygen and removal of waste products. Advanced QiGong practitioners can have an oxygen/carbon dioxide exchange rate ten times that of the average non-practitioner.

QiGong breathing by its nature, affects the heart and circulatory system. Not only does it provide a cleaner product (fully cleaned and oxygenated blood) but also regulates the flow of that product both by the physical movement of the body tissues and the mental movement of Qi.

In Chinese Medicine it is believed that the Lungs control Qi and that Qi controls blood. Regulated breathing thus controls both Qi and Blood.

Various emotional conditions obviously affect the process of breathing. When you are calm, your breathing is "normal". Regulating the breath can help balance the emotions which aids in calming the mind.

Three major methods of breathing are used in QiGong, Normal, Natural and Reverse.

Normal breathing refers to regulating the quality and duration of the breath. Normal breathing is used in the Buddha hands video.

In Natural breathing the lower abdomen expands with the inhale and contracts with the exhale. Some teachers recommend the expansion to include the whole area of the waist following the Belt Channel to stimulate both the Front-Lower Tan Tien and the Back-Ming Men.

In Reverse Breathing the lower abdomen contracts with the inhale and expands with the exhale. This is considered the highest form of breathing by some teachers.

Both encourage the breath to be deep, slow, even, and soft. Deep refers to breathing to or from the area just below the navel (Lower Tan Tien). It is very important to concentrate your focus just below the navel and not in the whole lower abdomen.

According to my teacher, if the whole lower abdomen is used an imbalance will occur in the Urinary Bladder which can result in the development of a fat lower abdomen and high blood pressure.

Inhaling causes the Qi to rise and contract—exhaling causes the Qi to sink and expand. It is best to breath through the nose. This warms the air and stimulates nerve endings in the nose that benefit many organs, tissues, and functions of the body including heart rate, blood pressure, and the respiratory muscles.

Some specific QiGong exercises require breathing through the mouth. The danger of breathing through the mouth is that the mouth has a direct link to the stomach. Opening that link brings the possibility of loosing digestive energy.

After a substantial period of deep regulated breathing there will be a gradual reduction in the amount of energy used in respiration which will further help the body relax.

Deep abdominal breathing massages the internal organs in the thorax and the abdomen and benefits the function of the cerebral cortex through the nerve reflexes.

2. REGULATING BODY

Regulating the body involves using posture to facilitate the flow of Qi within the body and /or receive and discharge Qi from outside the body more efficiently. Regulation of the body helps the mind to relax and relaxation of the mind helps the body to relax. During active relaxation, energy restoration in the body is promoted.

Particular body positions and/or movements cause specific manifestations of Qi flow in the body. This manifestation takes place both from the body position itself and the relative proximity of one part of the body to another.

When powerful energy centers(acupuncture points) pass other areas of the body they can induce Qi flow in those areas. This is especially true if there is a direct energetic connection between the two parts or if they have similar energetic qualities.

Rising postures cause the Qi to rise—lowering postures cause the Qi to sink—opening postures cause the Qi to disperse—closing postures cause the Qi to gather.

The holding of any posture causes some muscles to contract while other muscles relax. This causes various changes in the flow of Qi and Blood to various areas of the body which accounts for the efficacy of the posture.

3. REGULATING MIND

Regulating the mind is the most important of the three regulations. In fact, the other regulations already employ regulation of the mind.

SUBSTITUTE ONE THOUGHT FOR A THOUSAND THOUGHTS

Disease and stress create imbalance in the excitement/inhibition responses of our nervous system. Calming the mind with a single thought can produce a deep inhibitory state (rest) for the cerebral cortex. This offers the nervous system an opportunity to regulate its function and thereby improve our health. Often the therapeutic results of QiGong practice can be related to this phenomenon.

Qi follows the mind, therefore the mind can lead Qi. Leading the Qi with the mind is perhaps the most powerful aspect of QiGong. Body position, movement and breath all affect the flow of Qi in the body, but the mind is the single most important factor in directing Qi. The mind is unlimited. Focusing the mind on Qi or an acupoint can effect body physiology. The cerebrum supplies bio-electric energy to the tissues of the body. When the mind focuses on one area the dermal electricity increases in that area and decreases in surrounding tissues.

Some systems of QiGong require the practitioner to use the mind to lead Qi along a specific channel. This method is used to reinforce the flow of Qi in specific areas. Other systems require the practitioner to focus the mind on a distal area and expect the Qi to follow the natural course to that area. Both methods work and each has its strong and weak points.

The strong point of leading the Qi is that it will strongly augment the flow if the practitioner truly knows the course of the channel. The weak point is, of course, that if the exact channel pathway is not known the flow of Qi may actually be retarded.

The strong point of using a distal point of focus is that the Qi can follow its natural pathway. The weak point is that the Qi may not flow as powerfully.

For practitioners of Eighteen Buddha Hands, when advised by a competent Doctor, it is possible to focus the main emphasis of an appropriate exercise on a particular channel by either knowing and mentally leading the Qi along the course of that channel or by simply keeping the attention on the end point (or even the end finger or toe) of the correct channel.

TECHNIQUES

Techniques in this context does not refer to specific movements or exercises but to considerations both inside and outside the exercises themselves.

SITE

Choosing a quiet, pleasant and nurturing site will greatly enhance your practice. Some form of QiGong can be practiced almost anywhere and in later stages of development the practitioner will often practice throughout the routines of daily life.

The most important factor in location of the site is the availability of fresh air. Breath is one of the three regulations and air is an important source of energetic nutrition. One might say that you are what you breath.

Practicing in a forest, especially a pine forest, is ideal. Any area with lots of healthy greenery and low pollution is fine. Areas near oceans, lakes, or streams are also beneficial providing the atmosphere is not overly damp.

A modest knowledge of Feng Shui is invaluable in choosing a good practice area.

The ability to quiet your mind and ask yourself how you feel in a certain spot is important. Your body/mind/spirit will know whether a place "feels" right or not. For those who must practice indoors, seek a well ventilated room that you feel comfortable in and keep the room clean.

Gravesites are not auspicious places to practice, nor are areas with withered vegetation. Avoid extremes of heat, cold, wind, and damp. QiGong should not be practiced during heavy storms especially with thunder and lightning.

DIRECTION

There are many theories regarding the direction to face while practicing QiGong. As with site selection, one totally valid method is to quietly "feel" each direction and face the one in which you are most comfortable. You should feel outwardly stable and inwardly responsive as you quiet your mind and face the proper direction.

My teacher recommends facing the sun in the daytime and the moon at night.

Similar Qi's support and seek each other. South and East are considered Yang directions and North and West are considered Yin.

One school of thought suggests facing South or East to strengthen Yang and North or West to strengthen Yin. East relates to the wood element which represents growth. Since QiGong practitioners are attempting to grow their Qi, East is a popular direction to face especially in the morning as the sun (Yang) is rising.

Another school of thought looks at the front of the body as Yin and the back as Yang. Yin has sedating and downward qualities while Yang has tonifying and upward qualities. This school would face South and East to nourish Yin and face North and West to nourish Yang.

The directions are also associated with organs. East relates to the Liver- North to the Kidneys- South to the Heart- and West to the Lungs.

If one had weak Kidneys and excess Fire in the Heart which is common in chronic disease, he could face South.

The front of the body being Yin and facing South, the direction of the Heart which represents fire, would draw the Heart fire down. The back being Yang and facing North, the direction of the Kidneys, would bring Kidney energy up.

Using this theory a person with an excess Liver and deficient Lungs would face East. East is the direction of the Liver and the front of the body is Yin. The Liver excess would be brought down and the Lung energy would be brought up as the back of the body would face West.

With all these theories it may be difficult for the novice-or even an expert- to really know intellectually which direction is best. This brings us back to the "feeling" method which is simple and effective or simply following the sun or moon.

One last point concerning direction is that if an exercise moves to both left and right sides from the center and one begins to the right side the exercise is generally more tonifying while if one begins to the left side the exercise is generally more sedative in nature.

MOVEMENT

Upward movements make the Qi rise-downward movements make the Qi sink-opening movements spread Qi from the interior to the exterior-closing movements concentrate Qi from the extremities to the interior. These are the ways Qi is influenced by movement.

An excess of spreading will cause the Qi to dissipate and an excess of closing movements will cause the Qi to stagnate. Likewise,an excess of either upward or downward movements will cause imbalances in the re-spected direction of Qi flow.

Inhaling makes the Qi rise and concentrate while exhaling makes the Qi sink and spread to the extremities.

QiGong exercises use a combination of breath co-ordination and physical movement to regulate Qi flow in the desired manner, but the most important regulation is the mind.

In exercises requiring very powerful Qi flows, the mind, breath, and body movements may all co-ordinate to produce Qi flow in one direction. Often, in order to moderate Qi flow one of the three regulations may actually restrain the flow to create a better balance of Yin and Yang. For the same reason (balance) exercises are often performed on both the left and right sides.

When one body part, particularly if a potent acupuncture point is involved, moves past another body part or comes in close proximity to another part, the flow of Qi will be affected. The closer the distance and the closer the energetic connection between the two parts the greater the effect.

For instance raising your hand from foot to chest will cause Qi to rise in your body and lowering your hand from chest to foot will cause the Qi to sink. If your hand is closer to your body while rising than it is when descending the overall result of the two movements will be a rise in Qi (assuming your regulated mind wills the rise).

Often QiGong exercises contain more than one type of movement. The different types of movement restrain and promote each other, each being the prerequisite for the other. In these exercises breath, body movement and mind all modulate and harmonize each other to produce the desired effect. Systems of QiGong often have a variety of combinations.

Another type of movement that affects Qi in QiGong exercises involves the movement of soft-connective tissue. When muscles and tendons flex and contract over an acupuncture point, they activate the functions of that point. Depending on how many flexion/contraction cycles are performed the point will be either tonified, sedated or harmonized.

The Eighteen Buddha Hands QiGong requires eight repetitions of each movement which generally allows the function of the points to express themselves according to the body's needs.

Regarding the movements of air while breathing, long exhaling brings Qi down and reduces blood pressure by expanding blood vessels in the extremities while long inhaling brings Qi up and constricts blood vessels in the extremities.

People with excess conditions in the top and deficiency below should exhale longer than inhaling and of course those with upper deficiencies should inhale longer than exhaling.

Remember these are all general rules—

THE MIND IS THE MOST IMPORTANT REGULATOR!

In most cases the final step in any QiGong exercise should be to guide the Qi back to the Lower Tan Tien.

TIME

Spring and Summer are Yang seasons while Fall and Winter are considered Yin. It is easier to nourish Yang Qi in the Spring and Summer and to nourish Yin Qi in the Fall and Winter.

Morning is considered Yang and afternoon is considered Yin. It is easier to nourish Yang in the morning and Yin in the afternoon.

Generally in QiGong the morning is the best time to train because the Qi by nature is aroused and growing at that time.

Most systems of QiGong are balanced in such a way that training any time is appropriate.

TRAINING ANY TIME IS BETTER THAN NO TIME!

Environmentally the Qi is changing its yin/yang nature at sunrise, midday, sunset, and midnight. These are good times to train QiGong as the body can take advantage of the environmental changes to help make internal changes.

A "crest" of Qi moves through the twelve primary meridians in each twenty-four hour period spending two hours in each meridian system. If a practitioner has a disharmony in one of the meridian systems it is beneficial (if not convenient) to practice QiGong during the time of that system. The times are: Lung-3-5am Large Intestine-5-7am Stomach-7-9am Spleen-9-11am Heart 11am-1pm Small Intestine-1-3pm Urinary Bladder-3-5pm Kidney-5-7pm Pericardium-7-9pm Triple Burner-9-11pm Gall Bladder-11pm-1am Liver-1-3am.

For beginners it is advisable to practice QiGong once or twice a day for 20-40 minutes. One should not practice to the point of fatigue. With more experience the time can be lengthened to accommodate personal goals. Those with illnesses should seek the advice of a knowledgeable Doctor as to the duration and content of any exercise program.

ABSORBING ENERGY FROM NATURE

There are several important points on the human body where the internal energy of man can directly connect with the energy of the environment. These points are often used in QiGong practice to absorb supplemental energy from nature and to release excess or toxic energy from the body. These points will be discussed in detail in a later section.

COLOR

Color therapy can be used with QiGong practice. If the practitioner has a disharmony with one of his organ systems the color associated with that system can be utilized during daily practice. Any material of the appropriate color can be hung in view of the practitioner during practice. Viewing natural objects of the appropriate color is even better. Color therapy can be applied to the various 5-element strategies of Chinese Medicine but should not be attempted without the consultation of a knowledgeable Doctor.

Red is the color corresponding to the Heart, Small Intestine, Pericardium, and Triple Heater—Yellow is the color corresponding to the Spleen and Stomach—White is the color corresponding to the Lungs and Large Intestine, Black is the color corresponding to the Kidneys and Urinary Bladder—Green is the color corresponding to the Liver and Gall Bladder.

CHAPTER 3

QIGONG FOR SPIRITUAL DEVELOPMENT

The purpose of Spiritual QiGong from a Taoist point of view is to reach ENLIGHTENMENT, from a Christian point of view is to become ONE WITH GOD, from a Buddhist point of view is to reach BUDDHAHOOD, and from a Yoga point of view is to reach TRANSCENDENTAL UNION. All these terms refer to the same condition—singularity—the state beyond subject and object, yin and yang—beyond all duality. This is the goal of spiritual development.

The tools we have for evolving to this state are the body, mind and spirit. The techniques we have are our energetic practices whether they be called QiGong, Meditation, Yoga or Prayer.

As humans we all have certain obvious common physical features and less obvious common energetic/spiritual features.

If we decide to develop our gross physical bodies we can engage in a wide variety of physical disciplines such as weightlifting, swimming, calisthenics, etc. Each will develop our physical form somewhat differently depending on how it is done. However, there will be common benchmarks throughout the process. Our legs will get stronger, our arms will become more muscular, etc. If we recognize a lack of development in one area-due to our ignorance or our participation in an incomplete system-we can supplement that area with more exercises from our present discipline or with exercises from another discipline.

The same is true with our spiritual/energetic development. If we decide to develop our spiritual/energetic presence, we can engage in disciplines such as Yoga, Buddhist or Taoist QiGong, etc.

Each of these systems are complete in themselves, if the whole system is transmitted to the student. If for some reason the teacher is unable to transmit the whole system to the student it is sometimes possible to utilize parts of other systems to augment a partial system.

The techniques vary from discipline to discipline and each student is a unique individual so development will vary in some ways but there will be common benchmarks along the way.

These complete systems are designed to provide a path for the student to reach his goal. Because they evolved in different cultures, times, and places, each system places a unique emphasis on various aspects of the spiritual/ energetic body and uses its own terminology to describe the process of cultivation, but the goal is the same.

Seven Chakras

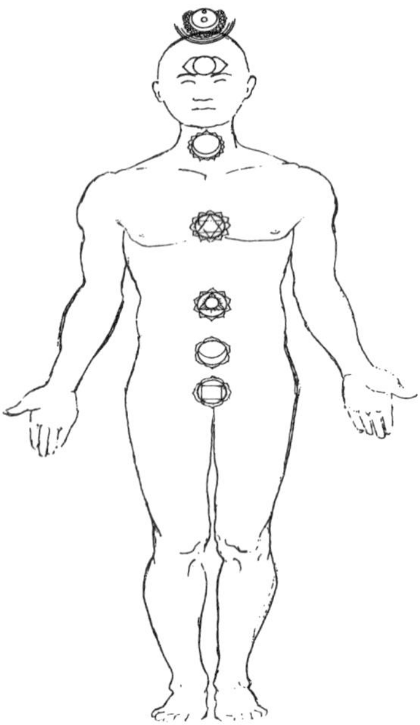

Buddhist and Yoga practitioners utilize three channels and seven Chakras (energy centers closely related to major nerve complexes) in their working models of major spiritual energetic structures and Taoists utilize three channels (somewhat different) three Tan Tiens (energy centers corresponding to three of the Chakras) and three treasures- Jing, Qi and Shen (Jing being the basic structural energy/matter of the body, Qi being the motive force of the body, and Shen being the Spirit that directs it all).

Three Tan Tiens

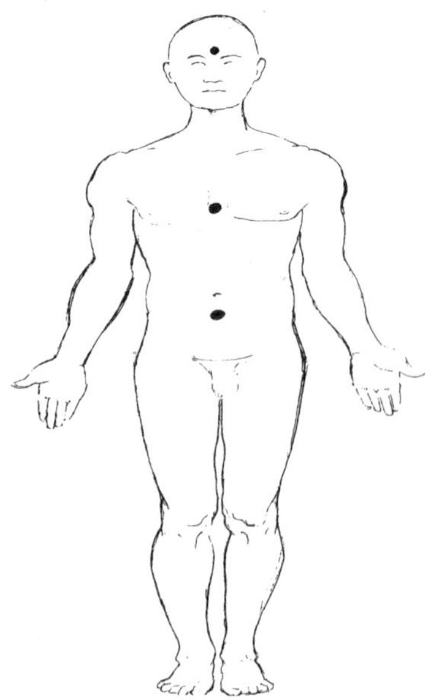

The channels that the Buddhist and Yoga practitioners use are the central channel (Sushumra) which runs up the middle of the spinal cord, the left side channel (Ida) which runs on the left side of the spine and the right side channel (Pingala) which runs on the right side of the spine.

These channels roughly begin at the base of the spine and meet in the Brow Chakra (Taoist Upper Tan Tien).

The left side channel is considered negative (Yin) and the right side channel is considered positive (Yang). The middle channel is neutral.

By harmonizing and invigorating the left side channel and the right side channel all three are opened and the latent Kundalini (an aspect of eternal supreme consciousness) begins to rise. Through disciplined practice the Kundalini rises up the spinal cord passing through each of the seven Chakras. Spiritual development (ultimately singularity) is reached through this process of Kundalini rising, purifying, energizing, and transforming each Chakra.

Some authorities view Kundalini as an Energy in itself and others view it as a blockage that is released when energy moves up the spine. In either case the primary principle is that energy does move up the spine to accomplish Spiritual transformation.

According to some authorities, the force that activates Kundalini is generated by the replacement of Apana-energy residing below the navel (Taoist Lower Tan Tien-water-residence of Jing) with Prana- energy residing in the chest (Taoist Middle Tan Tien-Fire-residence of Qi) with the aid of Agni-digestive fire (aspect of Taoist Ming Men).

Apana, which resides in the lower abdomen and controls the function of elimination, is considered to be overabundant in most people. An overabundance of Apana is detrimental to our health on physical, mental, and spiritual levels.

Prana, which is a generic name for cosmic energy as well as the name of the energy which resides in the chest in the human being,is considered deficient in most people. By replenishing Prana and removing excess Apana we improve our health and manifest our latent spiritual birthright.

Agni is cultivated to burn up the excess Apana and expedite the absorption of Prana.

Some authorities on Yoga do not emphasize the "replacement" theory. They often explain Energetic Transformation as the process of reversing the downward movement of Apana and the upward movement of Prana. The two energies meet and mix in Samana (the navel region). With help of Agni, an energetic reaction is then initiated which creates a greater potent energy that opens and rises in Sushumna (the Central Channel). This explanation directly parallels the Taoist view.

In conversations with Yoga practitioners, I am often asked where the left and right side channels are located in the Chinese Medical energetic model of the body. The channels are not shown on acupuncture charts nor are they mentioned in most translated literature that I am aware of.

In fact, there are two channels running upwards along the spine. They belong to Ming Men (*see page 11*) and as such definitely match the characteristics of the left and right channels. Although the channels are shown to begin in Ming Men and end in the tongue, their association with the Urinary Bladder Meridian can easily be used to fulfill the geographic requirements of the left and right channels.

It is my opinion that Ming Men and the Belt Channel have been greatly underplayed in the literature available in English on Taoist Cultivation.

Ming Men is the seat of energetic transformation for the whole body. Stimulating the Belt Channel to fill with Qi directly stimulates the Moving Qi between the Kidneys which accelerates the transformational energies of the whole body, especially the transformation of Jing to Qi.

The Ming Men Channels rise up from the Kidneys. The left Kidney is Yin (left side Channel) and the right Kidney is Yang (right side channel).

The three treasures Jing-yin, Qi-yang and Shen-neutral closely resemble the attributes of the Three Channels in Buddhist/Yoga model and move within the spine.

When the Kundalini becomes fully aroused (or opened depending on your view) the Three Channels become one as do the Three Treasures upon the completion of the transformation process of Taoist practices.

Taoist Cultivation closely resembles Buddhist/Yoga cultivation. The three channels Taoists use are the Governing Vessel which runs up the middle of the back from the perineum to the upper lip, the Conception Vessel which runs from the perineum to the chin on the front of the body and the Chong Mai which runs up the front of the body beside the Conception Vessel but has an internal branch that ascends the middle of the spinal cord (as does the Conception Vessel).

Actually the Taoists use all of the Extraordinary Vessels to generate and absorb more energy and to balance the transformation process.

In both Yogic and Taoist models, great heat is generated during the process of cultivation. The heat is useful, and in fact necessary, in its proper place but as with any fire care must be taken to assure that surrounding material is not scorched. If the proper safeguards are not taken the transformation process can actually be detrimental rather than liberating.

The Taoists utilize the Extraordinary Vessels to balance out any over heating. Other systems have other ways to accomplish this including highly complicated cleansing techniques.

The Taoist Three Treasures are Jing-the material foundation of life which resides in the lower Tan Tien just below and behind the navel (residence of apana for Buddhist/Yoga practitioners) and symbolized by water. Qi-the motive force of the body which resides in the Middle Tan Tien midway between and behind the nipples in the front of the body (residence of Prana for Buddhist/Yoga practitioners) and symbolized by fire...Shen-the controlling spirit of the body which resides in the Upper Tan Tien at the midpoint behind the eyebrows (meeting point of the Three Channels for Buddist/Yoga practitioners).

There are generally considered four stages of Taoist Cultivation.

REFINING JING AND CONVERTING IT TO QI—fusing Fire and Water-Prana and Apana

PURIFYING QI AND CONVERTING IT TO SHEN—circulating the refined product up the Chong Mai in the middle of the spine.

REFINE SHEN TO RETURN TO NOTHINGNESS—realization and direct experience of singularity.

CRUSHING NOTHINGNESS—Total Singularity.

From an intellectual point of view the Taoists mix the Fire (Prana) and Water (Apana), subject the mixture to the heat of Ming Men (Agni), and produce a refined substance which they circulate to manifest their latent Spiritual potential.

Historically practitioners of both Taoist and Buddhist/Yoga methods have reached transcendental states of singularity. Perhaps the intellectual differences are products of a consciousness so divorced from direct experience that in the end they are meaningless.

I once asked my Teacher what books I should read to get a better understanding of my Taoist Practices. His reply was that I should not read any books because they could only give me intellectual knowledge which was useless in the face of direct experience.

BODHIDHARMA-originator of the Eighteen Buddha Hands QiGong came to China from India. He was already highly developed when he arrived. Before he developed this system he spent nine years meditating "facing the wall". It is possible that he was exposed to Taoist Principles during his travels

As we shall see, the energetic construction of the Eighteen Buddha Hands QiGong utilizes the best of both Buddhist/Yoga and Taoist development models to provide the practitioner with an optimal internal environment for physical, mental, emotional, and spiritual development.

This discussion about Spiritual/Energetic development has been quite simplistic. There are many books on the market that give in-depth information regarding all aspects of this subject. The one aspect that cannot be presented in a book is of course DIRECT EXPERIENCE which places intellectual information in the realm of trivia.

CHAPTER 4

STRATEGIES FOR THE EIGHTEEN BUDDHA HANDS

Practicing the Eighteen Buddha Hands just the way they are presented in this book and the accompanying video, is the best and safest strategy. Unless under the direct care and with the advice of a qualified Doctor of Oriental Medicine with knowledge of QiGong nothing should be altered.

Eighteen Buddha Hands QiGong is a very balanced system. It utilizes the three regulations in such a manner that it can benefit any practitioner. In some systems there are beginning, intermediate, and advanced techniques, The Buddha Hands was ingeniously designed to facilitate development and provide a challenge for practitioners at all levels.

The highest theories of Chinese Medicine and the most subtle yet powerful energetic connections have been utilized in this system to provide for rapid yet safe development. Although Buddhist in origin, the lineage we practice is said to have been influenced by at least one Taoist Master.

Possible alternative strategies to be considered by a knowledgeable Doctor would primarily include altering the lengths of inhales or exhales to tonify or sedate yin or yang and to move the hands closer or further from the body to the same end. None of these changes should be made except on the advice of a knowledgeable Doctor.

If the whole set of exercises is not performed at one time the practitioner should ALWAYS COMPLETE WHOLE CHAPTERS. Each chapter is designed to bring specific balances to the practitioner and it is important to complete each Exercise in the chapter including the Standing Pose. Any number of chapters may be performed as long as all the exercises and the standing position following that chapter are completed.

If the practitioner lacks time or energy to complete the whole set, a knowledgeable Doctor can prescribe one or more chapters according to the practitioners condition and the overall theme of the individual chapters. Such choices require a solid knowledge of Oriental Medicine—which is beyond the scope of this book.

QiGong not only harmonizes the internal energies of man but also strengthens the link between man and nature so practicing outdoors in a pleasant setting is ideal.

The physical postures of the Eighteen Buddha Hands should be done in a relaxed manner, with as little physical tension as possible. The mind should lead the hands, which may be held in the appropriate position with a very gentle tension.

The body should move together, with all parts beginning each movement at the same time and ending the movement at the same time. Breath is coordinated with physical movement, beginning and ending with the movement unless otherwise instructed.

The lower spine should be slightly tucked (not locked) in to minimize the lower inward curvature of the spine which allows the Qi to move upwards in the spine more easily and stimulates Ming Men.

The top of the head should be gently lifted with the chin held slightly down and back to minimize the upper inward curvature of the neck which allows the Qi to move smoothly through the neck to the head.

The tip of the tongue should be held gently touching the roof of the mouth behind but not touching the teeth. This strengthens the connection between the Governing Vessel and the Conception vessel.

In some Yoga breathing exercises it is suggested that the tongue should be held on the floor of the mouth to avoid touching the teeth or roof of the mouth as this is believed to produce saliva and thereby disturb the mind. Yogic exercises usually do not utilize the Conception Vessel to return Qi back from the head as Taoist QiGong does.

Most Chinese systems believe saliva produced by QiGong is a valuable substance that should be collected and swallowed to the Lower Tan Tien. This saliva is said to aid digestion, supplement blood and body fluids, and nourish Essence.

The practitioner should wear loose clothing and flat shoes. Some styles of QiGong utilize a belt around the waist to help direct attention and Qi to the

Lower Tan Tien. In fact, many practitioners from the Shaolin Temple Lineage which is the lineage of the Eighteen Buddha Hands, use this technique. Unless the student is under the direct observation of a qualified teacher it is more advisable to keep the waist unencumbered.

It is not advisable to practice when you are in a hurry, tired, hungry, full, or emotionally upset. Usually training one hour after a meal and finishing one-half hour before a meal is appropriate.

Leading a regular balanced lifestyle with proper time for work, rest, and recreation will reinforce your practice and speed up results. A good diet and proper amounts of sleep are essential to progress.

During menstruation it is fine to practice but one should practice less vigorously and especially be gentle with exercises that tend to move the Qi downwards.

When one begins training QiGong, is advisable to abstain from sexual activity for a period of 100 days. Sexual energy is the basis of life and the transformational energy in the body. It is that energy QiGong seeks to nourish for better health and Spiritual Envolvement. This is especially important if one is training to heal some already apparent illness. After the 100 day period one should maintain moderate sexual activity.

Some common positive effects of training are increased warmth in the extremities, balanced appetite, increased intestinal peristalsis, deeper and more restful sleep, and an increase in saliva. Any excess saliva should be swallowed downwards to the lower Tan Tien as it is believed to be generated by Ming Men. This saliva is thought to be able to aid digestion, produce blood in the Heart, improve eyesight by replenishing the Liver, increase Qi in the Lungs and nourish Kidney essence. Often practitioners feel itching sensations on various areas of the body. This phenomenon means that the energy channels are being cleaned and opened at those areas. Crackling sounds in the joints and slight involuntary tremblings in the muscles indicate the Qi is moving with new force through the affected area. Quite soon after beginning practice of QiGong people often begin to notice their overall sense of well-being improve.

Dizziness, headache, fatigue, shortness of breath or tightness in the body, especially the shoulders are undesirable effects of training incorrectly. The cause of these undesirable effects is usually holding unnecessary tension in some part of the body--or mind. The method to correct these problems is to RELAX!

Following the descriptions of the exercises information regarding their effects on Body Systems, Primary Meridians, Extraordinary Vessels, Yin/ Yang Orientation, External\Internal implications, Acupuncture Points affected, and the Spiritual/Energetic Processes activated will be presented. There will also be a general commentary on each exercise.

Much of the information in this section is redundant and will not be repeated for every applicable instance. Also interest in some of the information will be limited to a small percentage of the readers. The information has been categorized to make it easy to find areas of interest and skip over less compelling areas.

Below is a brief explanation of each category.

BODY SYSTEMS

By definition QiGong "regulates the breath" so all QiGong affects the lungs (respiratory system). Since Qi is the commander of blood and QiGong, exercises control the Qi,the circulatory system will also be affected to some degree by all QiGong.

In Chinese Medicine, the Spleen is considered of primary importance in the digestive function and it also controls the Qi of the four limbs. Therefore, exercising the limbs will affect the digestive system.

Each Eighteen Buddha Hands moving exercise involves some movement of the body. When the body moves, pressure is exerted and released on the internal organs creating a pumping effect thereby stimulating the internal organs. In this section, we will mention the most obviously affected organ-systems for each exercise. Other systems will also be affected to a lesser degree.

PRIMARY MERIDIANS

Of the twelve Primary Channels six traverse the arms and six traverse the legs. As the arms or legs move in and out or up and down all the channels of the moving limb will be affected.

Certain movements are believed to affect specific meridians more than others. The effects are modified by the position or movement of the body, the direction of movement, and the relationship of body parts (especially the hands) to each other.

In this section we will point out the Primary Meridians directly affected by the exercise. Because of the many interconnections of the Qi pathways of the body other aspects of the system will also be affected. In fact, as the practitioner becomes more advanced and "open" inside, any movement (including movement of the mind-thought) will begin to affect a larger number of pathways.

A thorough study of the energetic physiology of the body according to Chinese Medicine will reveal the more subtle connections to the interested student.

EIGHT EXTRAORDINARY VESSELS

Each exercise in this system also directly affects one or more of the Extra-Ordinary Vessels and of course indirectly affects others. These Vessels are affected either through the body position or movement. Often the controlling points-master points- of the Vessels are directly stimulated.

YIN/YANG

The exercises of Eighteen Buddha Hands accent either Yin Qi ,Yang Qi or Balance. Depending on the regulations of the practitioner, the exercises can be used therapeutically to address specific Yin/Yang imbalances. Defensive energy in the body is considered Yang and nutritive energy is considered Yin.

EXTERNAL/ INTERNAL

Each exercise has an inherent internal\external affiliation. In other words, some exercises by design and mental focus address circulation within the body and others allow for a direct communication with nature.

ACUPUNCTURE POINTS

Acupoints regulate Qi flows in the body, open channels, and communicate with the external environment. Each exercise in this system stimulates many acupoints of which we will discuss several of the most important.

It is suggested that the reader consult the acupuncture point reference section in the back of the book to get a more detailed understanding of the full implications of each exercise.

For health practitioners the point section should be a starting place to do further research to better prescribe various exercises for your patients.

In general, the acupuncture points affected by these exercises increase the flow of Qi, remove toxins, strengthen the immune system and open the Extra-Ordinary Vessels.

SPIRITUAL/ENERGETIC PROCESSES

Spiritual development can be seen as the work of balancing the Qi of the whole body, cultivating and refining Qi, enhancing communication between the three Tan Tiens, and ultimately reaching singularity. This is accomplished through utilizing the Qi Channels of the body-especially the Extra-Ordinary Vessels-with the three regulations to systematically unlock our latent birthright. This section will explain which parts of that process individual exercises and chapters facilitate.

BREATHING TECHNIQUES

There are several breathing patterns appropriate to the 18 Hands QiGong. Among these patterns are Normal Breathing, Natural Breathing and Reverse Breathing.

In Normal Breathing the breath is regulated in volume and length but not in destination.

In Natural Breathing the breath is regulated in volume, length and destination. The destination is the lower abdomen (Tan Tien). Upon inhalation, the lower abdomen is expanded and upon exhalation, the lower abdomen is contracted. This method is widely used in Yoga "Pranayama" exercises and many Buddist practices.

In Reverse Breathing the breath is regulated in volume, length and destination. The destination is also the lower abdomen but in this case, the lower abdomen is contracted upon inhaling and expanded during the exhale. This is sometimes called the Toaist Breathing as the technique is common among Toaist practitioners. Many authorities consider Reverse Breathing the most advanced of the three methods.

The 18 Buddha Hands QiGong Video utilizes Normal Breathing as it is the easiest and the safest method. Normal Breathing allows the positions and movements of the body to regulate the destination of the breath.

Both Natural and Reverse Breathing techniques should be used only with the guidance of a qualified QiGong Teacher.

For the information purposes of this book, Reverse Breathing will be explained with the exercises. Upon inhalation, the lower abdomen will contract and the breath will usually be directed either to the Middle Tan Tien (chest) or the Ming Men (located directly behind the navel at the spine). Exhaling will involve expanding the lower abdomen and directing the breath to the Lower Tan Tien (just below the navel).

The explanations in this book are not the only breathing techniques that can be used with Buddha Hands.

REMEMBER-USE ONLY NORMAL BREATHING UNLESS GUIDED BY A QUALIFIED QIGONG MASTER.

CHAPTER 5

EIGHTEEN BUDDHA HANDS QIGONG

CHAPTER ONE
IMMORTAL SALUTES WITH FOLDED HANDS

An Immortal is a being of high Spiritual development, which is a Yang state. Saluting infers deference to a higher power. In this case, the reference may be to the folded hands which preclude direct communication with the highest Yang-Heaven. Even in the standing position at the end of this chapter direct communication between Heaven and Earth is modulated by the fingers of the open hands facing each other.

Exercise One

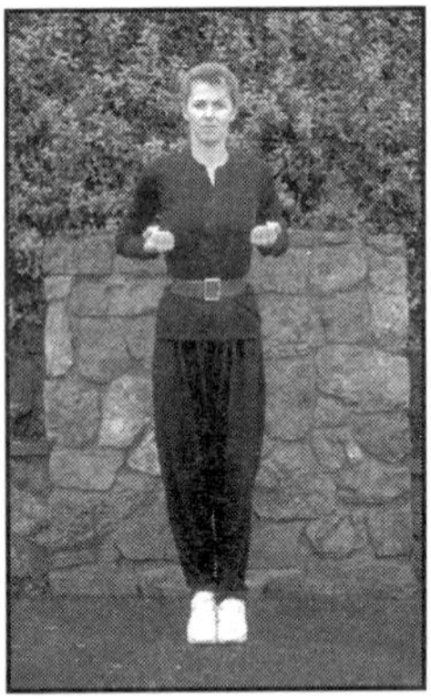

One A

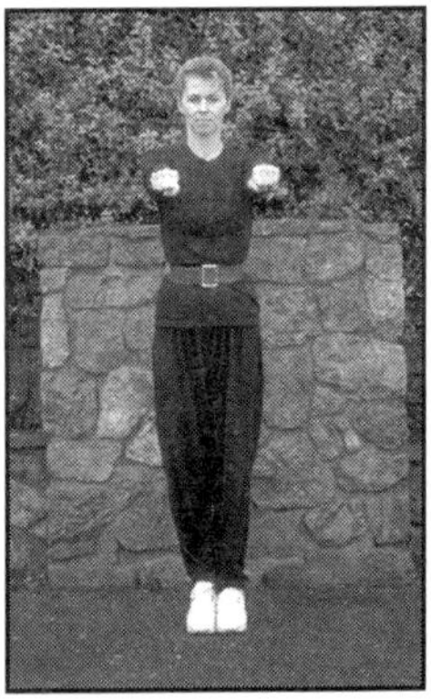

One B

Stand with the feet together and arms hanging naturally at the sides.

Slowly form the hands into fists with the palms facing upwards and raise both fists along the sides of the body as high as comfortably possible, inhaling to the chest with the lower abdomen contracted as in figure **One A.**

Extend both fists away from the body parallel to the ground while gradually turning the palms downward and exhaling to the Lower Tan Tien as in figure **One B.**

As the fists reach full extension open the hands with the palms facing forward and the fingers pointing straight up. Rotate the open palms laterally until the fingers point downward. At this point, form fists with the hands and return the fists to the sides of the body while inhaling to the chest.

Perform this extension while exhaling-revolve palms-retraction while inhaling movement eight times.

The revolving palm motion is often used in the 18 Buddha Hands Exercises as a transition between one movement and another. While performing this revolving maneuver, the first half of the movement is always done while still exhaling and the second half is done while beginning the inhale.

At the end of the eighth repetition you should be in the position of figure **One A** with your lungs full of air.

Exhale.

BODY SYSTEMS
Respiratory System, Circulatory System

PRIMARY CHANNELS
Lung, Large Intestine, Pericardium, Triple Heater, Heart, Small Intestine

EXTRAORDINARY VESSELS
Governing Vessel, Conception Vessel Chong Mai, Yin Chiao Mai, Yin Wei Mai, Yang Wei Mai

YIN/YANG ORIENTATION
Yang In this exercise the body is held upright with the feet together which is a Yang standing position. The arm movements are confined to the upper part of the body with no downward motions and therefore, the arms do not modulate the Yang body position with downward motions. The arm movements are somewhat neutral in that they remain parallel to the ground. If they rose it would accent the Yang nature of the exercise and if they dropped it would accent the Yin nature of the exercise.

EXTERNAL/INTERNAL ASPECTS
Internal Throughout the exercise the hands are kept in fists except at the

arms extended position where the hands open to perform the clawing motion before returning. Keeping the hands in fists helps to retain the flow of Qi within the body.

On the upper limb, Pericardium 8 is the major point of communication between the inside Qi and the environmental Qi. With the hands in fists that communication is muted. Without special regulation of the mind the Qi of the body will seek to harmonize itself throughout the clawing motion. If there is excess or toxic energy in the body, it can dissipate and if there is deficiency extra Qi from the environment, it can be assimilated. By regulating the mind, the practitioner can accent either gathering or releasing during the clawing motion. The releasing of energy should coincide with the ending of the exhale cycle and the gathering should coincide with the beginning of the inhale cycle.

ACUPUNCTURE POINTS
LI4, SI3, LU7, LU9, TB4, SP4, Ki6, CV17, GV14, P6, P7, P8, HE7

In the standing position both KI6 and SP4 are brought into close proximity to each other and are thereby mildly stimulated. These are the Master points of Yin Chiao Mai and Chong Mai. When the fists are positioned beside the chest, the chest is expanded and CV17 is opened. CV17 is the meeting point to the Qi of the entire body. When the fists are fully extended, the upper back is expanded and GV14 is opened. GV14 is the point at which all the Yang Meridians of the body meet. By fully extending the little finger and thumb during the clawing motion LI4, SI3 and LU7,9 are opened. LI4 is one of the most important points on the body for expelling external pathogenic conditions and strengthening and regulating defensive Qi. SI3 is the master point of the Governing Vessels and LU7 is the Master Point of the Conception Vessels. LU9 is the reunion point of all the blood vessels of the body i.e. the main point that influences the Qi that moves the blood throughout the body. By fully spreading the palms and bending the wrists backward as close to ninety degrees as possible P6, P7, P8, HE7, TB4 and TB5 are stimulated. P6 is the Master Point of Yin Wei Mai and TB5 is the Master Point of Yang Wei Mai. P8 is the main point for connecting the Qi of man with the Qi of nature on the upper limb. TB4 is the Source point of the Triple Burner.The Triple Burner distributes Source Qi from the Kidney/ Ming Men complex to the Twelve Primary Meridians, each of which has a Source point to directly communicate with Source Qi. The Source point of the Triple Burner- Envoy of Source Qi- has a powerful strengthening effect on Source Qi. TB4 is particularly used in the Japanese Acupuncture Tradition, typically with a Gold Needle,for strengthening Source Qi. Both P7 and HE7 are Source points of their respective Meridians and are major points to regulate the Heart and to restore peace and harmony to the Spirit.

SPIRITUAL/ENERGETIC PROCESS

The Governing Vessel and Conception Vessel are very directly opened in this exercise through their Master Points. The Taoist Practice of opening and circulating Qi through these two Vessels is called the Microcosmic Orbit. Successful attainment of the Microcosmic Orbit Practice involves refining Jing (stored in Kidney) and converting it to Qi. This refined Qi is circulated through the two vessels and finally led to the head to nourish the Shen. Because these two Vessels control all the Yin and Yang of the body they are of the greatest importance to the general health of the body, which supports Spiritual Development.

The Microcosmic Orbit

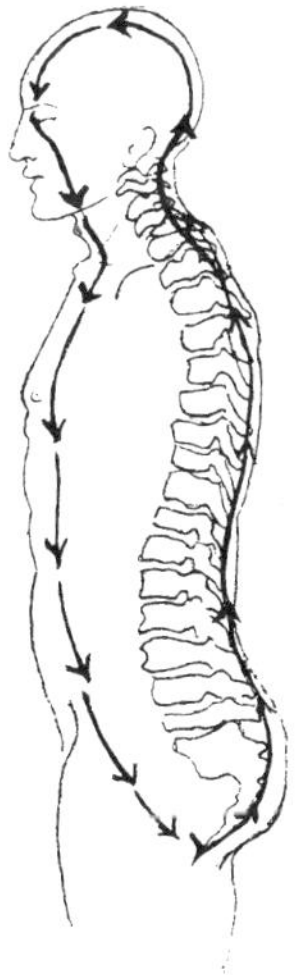

Successful Microcosmic Orbit Practice is not as easily attained as we might think. Of course there is Qi flowing in all the channels all the time and through various exercises it is possible to feel unusual sensations along the courses of the channels. An unusual sensation does not necessarily mean that refined Jing is flitting about through your channels. Radiation of sensation along a channel is common in many therapeutic techniques. Real refinement comes from many years of training a good system in the correct way. Some authorities believe that when the Conception Vessel truly "OPENS" the Chong Mai (Central Channel) will automatically open. The Governing Vessel, Conception Vessel and Chong Mai all originate from the same place. It is interesting to note that the internal branch of the Chong Mai, which is the branch most associated with Spiritual Development, and the internal branch of the Conception Vessel, both ascend the inside of the spinal column. Both are said to contain blood, Jing and both flow up the body to the face on their ventral branches .

The Master Point of Chong Mai is stimulated by body position in this exercise, as is the Master Point of Yin Wei Mai. The Yin Wei Mai is coupled with Chong Mai in Chinese Medicine. It actually connects the Yin channels of the arms and legs to the Conception Vessel and has a special relationship with the Heart. P6, Master Point of Yin Wei Mai, is often used for emotional problems and calming the Spirit in the practice of Acupuncture.

The Yin Heel Channel is quite important in QiGong practice. One of its main sources of Qi is from the conversion of Jing to Qi. It also gathers essence from the sexual organs and due to its master point sharing the Kidney Meridian with Ki1 it is well situated to gather energy from the earth.

The Yin Heel Channel runs up the Yin portion of the body to the brain. It is a major source of nourishment for the Spirit. The Yang Wei Mai links the Yang Channels of the hands and feet to the Governing Vessel. Its main sphere of influence is the exterior, defensive energy of the body. Defense of the body is important for health and spiritual work.

COMMENTARY

As the fists are raised to the sides of the chest while inhaling to the Middle Tan Tien, the Qi from the Lower Tan Tien is joined with the Qi of the Middle Tan Tan Tien-Water meets Fire. This motion also activates the function of all three burners, thereby mobilizing the whole organ system. As the hands are pushed out while exhaling to the lower Tan Tien, the Qi is sunk to the Lower Tan Tien where the Fire and Water can mix and transform.

At the same time Qi from the Lower Tan Tien moves out to the extremities. After the clawing motion in which Qi could have been exchanged with the environment if needed, the fists are drawn back to the sides of the chest while inhaling to the Middle Tan Tien. The Qi is collected back to the chest from the extremities and the lower Tan Tien. The cycle continues.

This predominantly Yang exercise has a strong influence on the defensive energy of the body. The Governing Vessel, Conception Vessel, and Chong Mai all carry Defensive Qi and most of the Acupuncture points directly stimulated function to expel external pathogenic influences and/or strengthen the defensive and supporting energies of the body.

Exercise Two

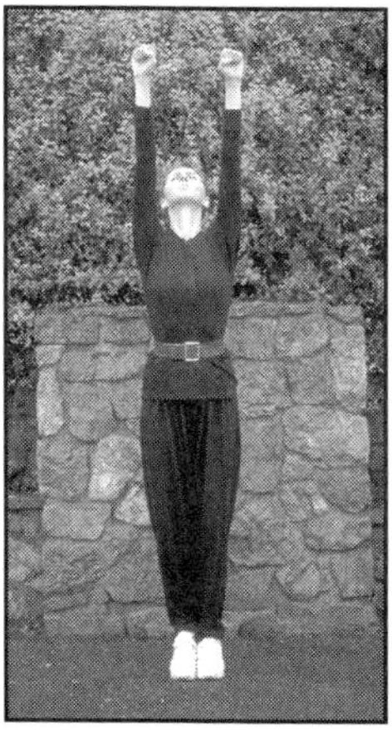

One C

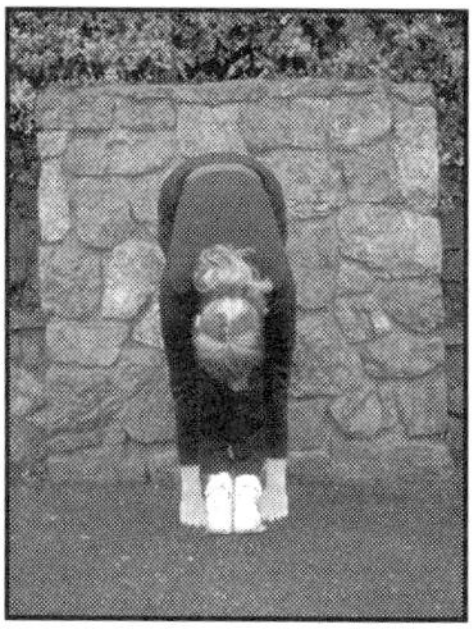

One D

Raise both fists overhead with the palms gradually turning to face forward while inhaling to the chest and contracting the lower abdomen as in figure **One C.**

Bend at the waist and extend the fists downward close to the body until they reach the ground in front of the toes exhaling to the Lower Tan Tien as in figure **One D**.

When the fists reach the ground perform the revolving hands motion again beginning to inhale half way through the movement.

Now raise the fists close to your body and begin to straighten your waist as you inhale to the chest. The palms will face upwards until they reach the chest when they will gradually turn forwards until they reach the position of figure **One C** again.

Repeat this sequence from figure **One C** to **One D**, revolve hands and return to figure One C eight times, inhaling to the chest on the way up and exhaling to the lower abdomen on the way down.

At the end of the eighth repetition you should be in the position shown in figure **One C** with your lungs full of air.

Exhale.

BODY SYSTEMS
Respiratory System, Circulatory System, Genito-urinary System, Digestive System

PRIMARY CHANNELS
Lung, Large Intestine, Heart, Small Intestine, Pericardium, Triple Heater, Urinary Bladder,Stomach.

EXTRA-ORDINARY VESSELS
Governing Vessel, Conception Vessel, Chong Mai, Yin Chiao Mai, Yin Wei Mai, Yang Wei Mai, Belt Channel.

YIN/YANG ORIENTATION
Yang In this exercise the body position with feet together and arms reaching upwards is a Yang position and the bent over position is Yin. With the proper mind and breath regulation this exercise could accent either Yin or Yang. The final consideration in the form is the amount of movement. A large movement tends to be Yang while a small movement is more Yin. In this case the movement is large which adds a Yang accent to the overall exercise. This exercise, under the proper guidance, can be used to bring excess Yang down.

EXTERNAL-INTERNAL
Internal As in the first exercise of this chapter, the hands are kept in fists throughout the exercise except for the clawing motion. In this case, the clawing motion is performed with hands facing the ground. This offers the opportunity to connect with the Yin energy of the ground and draw it upwards with mind regulation. This will balance the Yang nature of the exercise and also brings a more external aspect to the exercise. Without that effort of Mind Regulation, the external exposure is minimal.

ACUPUNCTURE POINTS
LI4, SI3, LU7, LU9, TB4, TB5, SP4, KI6, CV17, GV14, P6, P7, P8, HE7
See descriptions in Exercise One CV6, UB23, GV4

In this exercise it is the raising of the hands over the head that opens CV17 and the lowering of the hands to the feet that opens GV14. Lowering the hands while exhaling is a technique for ridding the body of turbid Qi, which supports the cleansing functions of this exercise.

CV6, GV4, and UB23 are all stimulated by the action of bending and raising the body at the waist. CV6 also called the Sea of Qi and Tan Tien, is in fact the front door to the Tan Tien, storehouse of the Postnatal and Prenatal Qi. It is considered the energetic center of the body, capable of tonifying Source Qi, Yang Qi, and Blood while nourishing Yin Qi. GV4 also called Ming Men is the back door to the Tan Tien and the point most able to directly access the Moving Qi between the Kidneys—Ming Men. UB23 is a point of direct access to the Kidneys. It is also capable of tonifying Source Qi, Qi, and Essence and nourishing Kidney Yin. All three of these points are intimately connected in the storage and transformative functions so necessary for good health and Spiritual /Energetic development.

SPIRITUAL/ENERGETIC PROCESS

This exercise utilizes the same points as exercise one to augment Spiritual / Energetic development with the addition of the bending motion. The act of bending forward at the waist and returning stimulates the Conception Vessel, Governing Vessel and Chong Mai. The extra stretch of having the arms overhead and the hands pushed to the feet adds to this effect. When Chong Mai actually opens, it is said that one experiences the feeling of an infinite extension from the head up and the feet down. Stretching the body,as this exercise does, encourages that feeling inside the body and aids that development. The waist motion also brings into play the Belt Channel, GV4, CV6, and UB23 with all their tonic, transformative and storing qualities.

COMMENTARY

Raising the hands overhead while inhaling to the chest brings the Lower Tan Tien Qi up to meet the Qi of the Middle Tan Tien and lowering the hands to the feet while exhaling brings the Middle Tan Tien Qi down to mix with that of the Lower Tan Tien—Fire and Water communicating. The action of the waist bending brings into play the transforming energies of the Ming Men through the action of GV4 and stimulation of the Belt Channel. This mechanical process also increases the stimulation of the Governing Vessel, Conception Vessel, and Chong Mai. Here the mixing of Fire and Water is augmented with the activation of the transformative energies to initiate the Jing to Qi alchemical process. By looking up when the hands are raised, energy is stored in the Kidneys rather than allowed to circulate in the Microcosmic Orbit. The first exercise pertains more to the Middle Tan Tien and this exercise links the Lower and Middle Tan Tiens while emphasizing the storage and transformative qualities of the Lower Tan Tien.

Standing

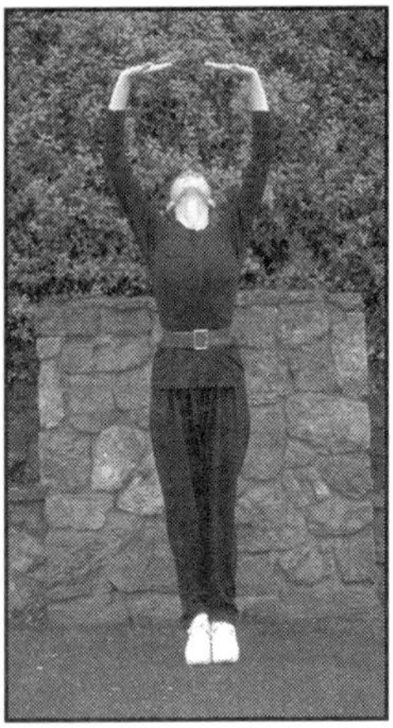

One E

From figure **One D** open your fists, point your middle fingertips at each other and face your palms upwards. Look straight up and breath naturally as in figure **One E.**

Hold this position for eight breaths.

When finished stand naturally and wait until your breath returns to normal before going on to the second chapter.

BODY SYSTEMS
Respiratory System, Circulatory System, Digestive System

PRIMARY CHANNELS
Lung, Large Intestine, Heart, Small Intestine, Pericardium Triple Heater

YIN/YANG
Yang

EXTERNAL/INTERNAL
External The open palms link Man and Heaven

ACUPUNCTURE POINTS

P8, P9, TB4, TB5, LI4, HE7, P6, P7, LU7, LU9, SP4, KI6, SI3 see previous exercise—P9 is the main point not seen in the moving exercises of this chapter. P9, being on the tip of the middle finger, is the most distal point on the upper limb. It has a very close connection with the Heart. When the P9 points of both hands are in close proximity the energetic circle formed by the two arms and the Middle Tan Tien is activated.

SPIRITUAL/ENERGETIC PROCESS

The Master Points of the Governing Vessel are opened by this pose, but the Vessel is mechanically closed by the position of the head. The Master Points of Chong Mai are opened by their proximity to each other and flow is encouraged in the Channel by the extended position of the body. The same is true with the Yin Chaio Mai. As the Governing Vessel is contracted closed, the Conception Vessel is stretched open and stimulated by the opening of its Master Points through the stretching of the hands.

Yin Wei Mai (Master Point P6-Inner Gate) and Yang Wei Mai (Master Point TB5-Outer Pass) are stimulated by their respective Master Points and by the energetic exchange of internal/external Qi.

One of the functions of the Kidneys is to anchor the air inhaled through the Lungs. This position allows the body to gather the Yang Qi of Heaven and to a lesser degree the Yin Qi from Earth and store both in the Kidneys.

COMMENTARY

The standing position with arms raised and legs straight is a Yang Position. The open hands allow the communication of the internal Qi with Heaven Qi, but the fingers of the open hands are pointed at each other. At each of the three Tan Tiens there is a circular energy pattern within the body. Holding the arms extended in a circle with the fingers pointing at each other activates and emphasizes the circular pattern of the Middle Tan Tien. The standing position requires the head be held up facing Heaven. This as we have already seen causes the storage function of the Kidneys to be activated and shuts off the circulation in the Microcosmic Orbit. With the hands held palms up and fingers facing each other, the Qi of Heaven and Man can communicate through the Middle Tan Tien. The face is also an important exchange area for the Qi of man and the environment. The face contains the sense organs of the eyes, ears nose, and mouth. Although each of these sense organs is associated with an internal organ, the overall information gathered is processed by the mind-Heart- Middle Tan Tien. The Qi of Heaven is considered Yang Qi, so we have a large amount of Yang Qi converging in the Middle Tan Tien.

A Yang position will tend to make Qi rise in the body. Just by the position alone some Yin Qi will be drawn upwards from the Earth through Ki1 during the inhale.

Breathing naturally with a quiet mind will allow the Qi of Heaven and Earth to harmonize with an emphasis on gathering the Qi of Heaven in the Middle Tan Tien, opening the Heart to Divine Grace.

CHAPTER TWO *WARRIOR KING LEFTS THE CAULDRON*

Eighteen Buddha Hands QiGong originated in Shaolin Temple. Supposedly when a man completed the training at the temple, one of the final test was to lift a hot cauldron using the forearms. The cauldron was so hot that the symbols on the sides where the forearms touched were burned onto the arms of the student. These symbols were a Dragon and a Tiger. A graduate of Shaolin could be recognized by the scarred symbols left on his arms which signified great strength of body, mind, and Spirit. This chapter more than any other has the potential of building strength. The second exercise in this chapter has been used as the physical exercise for developing the Iron Palm. In this method, the hands were thrust into various mixtures of heated herbs and iron filings.

Exercise One

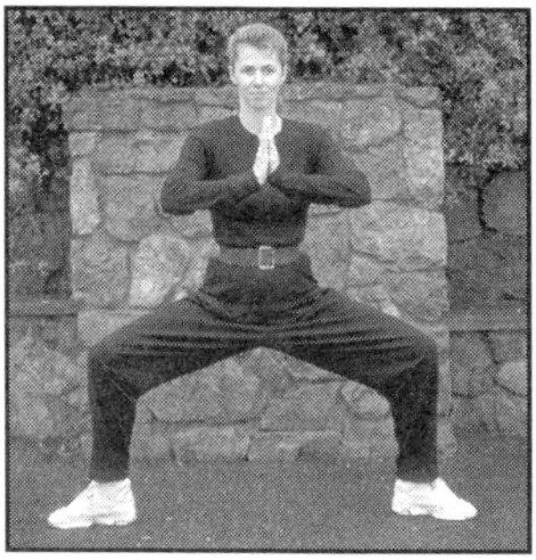

Two A

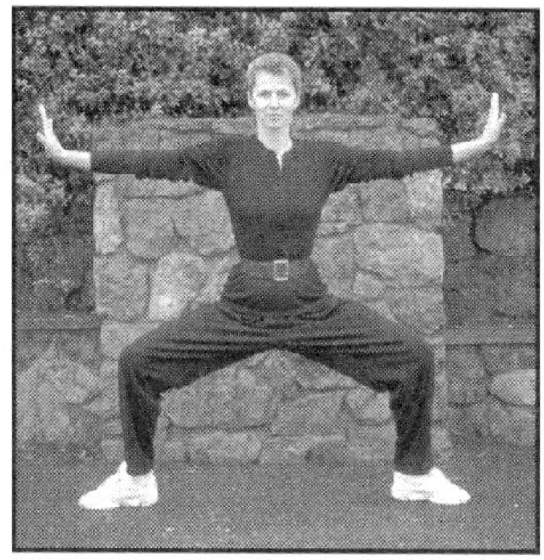

Two B

Spread the feet wide apart forming a toe-heel-heel-toe straight line and bending the knees as in figure **Two A**. Gently join the palms in front of the chest with fingers pointing up.

Spread both palms forward and outward towards the sides inhaling to the chest as in figure **Two B**.

When the palms reach full extension to the sides return them along the same pathway to the position in figure **Two A** exhaling to the lower abdomen.

Repeat this spreading-inhaling and retracting-exhaling motion eight times.

At the end of the eighth repetition you will be in position Two A with the lungs empty.

BODY SYSTEMS
Respiratory System, Circulatory System

PRIMARY CHANNELS
Lung, Large Intestine, Heart, Small Intestine, Pericardium, Triple Heater—The position of the legs opens all the Yin Channels of the legs-Spleen, Liver, and Kidney while tending to close the Yang Channels.

YIN/YANG ORIENTATION
This exercise is primarily Yin in nature. The knees are deeply bent and the

feet turned out to the point of forming a straight line. This opens all the Yin channels of the legs and tends to close the Yang channels. The arms are spreading out and back at the level of the upper body which is a Yang position, but they are functioning as a pump to draw Yin upwards.

EXTRA-ORDINARY VESSELS
Governing Vessel, Conception Vessel, Yin Wei Mai, Yang Wei Mai, Yin Chiao Mai, Chong Mai.

INTERNAL/EXTERNAL
External In this exercise the palms (P8) are spread and exposed throughout.

ACUPUNCTURE POINTS
SI3, P8, P7, P6, LU7, LU9, TB4, TB5, HE7, CV17, GV14, SP4, KI6
SP4 and Ki6 Master points of Chong Mai and Yin Chiao Mai are opened by the spreading of the feet to the sides. P8, the major point of communication between man and nature on the upper extremities, is opened by the spreading palms and hand position as are the points SI3, P6, P7, LU7, LU9, TB4, TB5, HE7, CV17, and GV14. SI3 is the Master Point of the Governing Vessel, P6 is the Master Point of Yin Wei Mai, LU7 is the Master Point of the Conception Vessel, TB5 is the Master Point of Yang Wei Mai, P7 and HE7 are points that regulate the Heart and bring Peace and Harmony to the Spirit. LU9 is the reunion point of the energy that moves the blood in the vessels of the entire body, GV14 is the meeting point of all the Yang Channels in the body and a major point to strengthen defensive energy, and CV17 is the meeting point of the Qi of the body.

SPIRITUAL/ENERGETIC PROCESS
The beginning position with palms together increases the flow and concentration of Qi in the Middle Tan Tien, regulates the Heart, and calms the Spirit. Some styles of QiGong feel that the position of palms touching is so powerful that it is not incorporated in their exercises until an advanced stage. As the palms spread to the side and the practitioner inhales to the chest, Qi from the Earth is drawn upwards through Ki1 and the open Yin Channels to the Middle Tan Tien. At the same time, Qi from the environment is drawn in through the palms to the Middle Tan Tien.

As the palms are drawn together while exhaling, the Qi collected in the Middle Tan Tien is concentrated in the Lower Tan Tien. In some traditions, Qi drawn from the earth is directed to Ming Men and Qi drawn from the environment is directed to CV15, the Luo point of the Conception Vessel where Yin Qi is said to descend from the chest. The mental regulation calls for descending the Qi back to the Lower Tan Tien for storage . The important point is, as always, MIND REGULATION.

Here again we have a mixing of Qi-Fire from the Middle Tan Tien and Jing-Water from the Lower Tan Tien. The opening and closing movements pump the Governing Vessel and the Conception Vessel and the rising and falling of the Qi stimulate the Chong Mai. Internal and external Qi are harmonized by the opening of Yin and Yang Wei Mai. Inhaling up to the chest and exhaling down to the Lower TanTien always has a mild pumping effect on the CV6-GV4 axis so the transformative and storage functions to Ming Men-Tan Tien are stimulated.

COMMENTARY
This exercise is well suited to accenting any one of the channels of the arm by concentrating mind on either the course of the channel or the distal point-digit of the channel. Generally these further mind regulations are not necessary as the Qi is intelligent in its own right and will seek to balance itself once it is mobilized.

Exercise Two

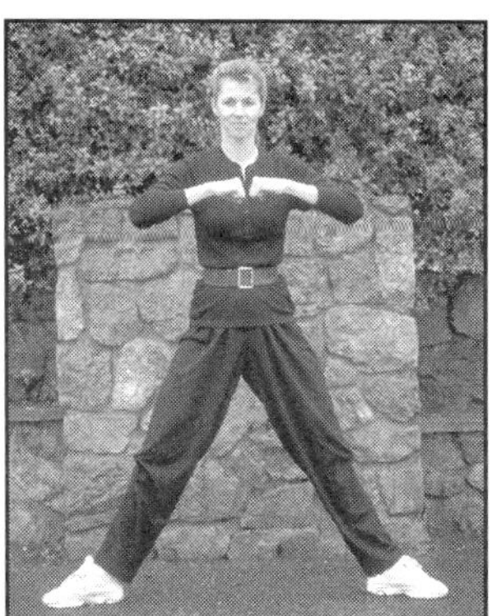

Two C

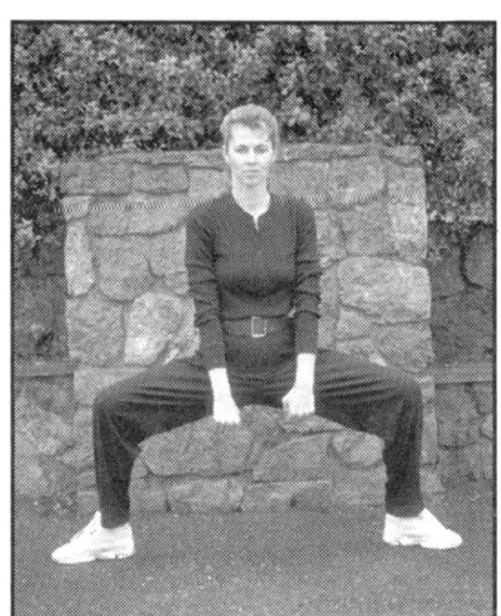

Two D

Form fists with the hands, raise the forearms to a position parallel to the ground with palms facing down, and stand upright while inhaling to the chest as in figure **Two C**.

Bend the knees and extend the fists downwards with the palms facing the body exhaling to the lower abdomen as in figure **Two D**.

At the full downward extension perform the revolving hands with palms facing the ground and return to position **Two C** while inhaling to the chest.

Repeat this upward-inhaling and downward-exhaling movement eight times.

At the end of the eighth repetition you will be in the position shown in figure **Two D** with your lungs empty.

BODY SYSTEMS
Respiratory System, Circulatory System, Digestive System

PRIMARY CHANNELS
All the Primary Channels of arms and legs are pumped during this exercise.

EXTRA-ORDINARY VESSELS
Governing Vessel, Conception Vessel. Yin Wei Mai, Yang Wei Mai, Chong Mai, Yin Chiao Mai

YIN/YANG ORIENTATION
Yin—This exercise begins from a Yin standing position. There is a fair amount of movement of the body which tends to develop Yang but the mind regulation fosters Yin. The arms never move above the chest-where all the Yin Primary Channels end.

EXTERNAL/INTERNAL
This exercise can be classed both internal and external because the palms are closed throughout but the mental regulation strongly induces gathering Qi from the Earth.

ACUPUNCTURE POINTS
Same as Chapter 2 Exercise One. In this case P8 is used to gather Qi from the Earth or release turbid Qi into the Earth.

SPIRITUAL/ENERGETIC PROCESS

The up and down movements stimulate The Governing Vessel, Conception Vessel, Chong Mai and Yin Chiao Mai. Yang Chiao Mai, even though the body position tends to render it closed, will receive some stimulation through up and down movements. Since the hands stop at the chest, the functions of all the Vessels will be modulated to favor communication between the Middle Tan Tien and the Lower Tan Tien-gathering Yin Qi from Earth, raising it to meet with Fire Qi from the Middle Tan Tien, and returning the mixture to the Lower Tan Tien for transformational activity. This transformational activity will be driven by Ming Men which is activated by the breath.

COMMENTARY

This exercise is extremely powerful because the Three Regulations are all co-ordinated in the same direction-moving upward, inhaling upward, and thinking upward—moving downwards, exhaling downwards, and thinking downwards. In Chinese Martial Arts, physical power is directly reciprocal to the connection with Earth. This exercise offers unlimited connection with Earth.

Standing

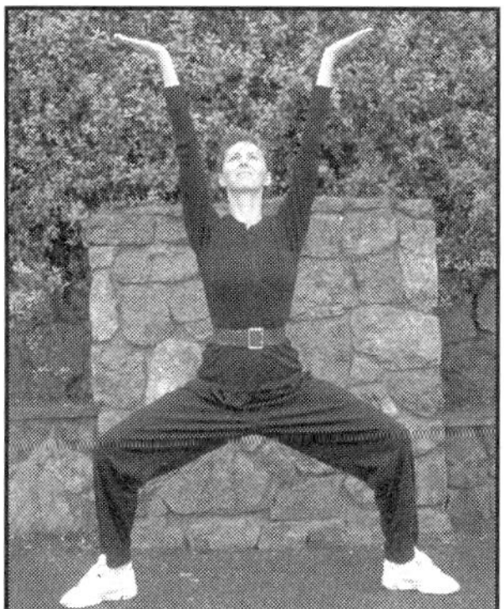

Two E

While breathing normally raise your open palms upward with the fingers pointing laterally as in figure **Two E**. Look slightly upwards. Hold this position for eight breaths.

BODY SYSTEMS
Respiratory, Circulatory, Digestive—Raising of the arms overhead extends the vertical range of the diaphragm which increases depth of respiration and provides an internal massage for the digestive organs and Heart.

PRIMARY CHANNELS
All

EXTRA-ORDINARY VESSELS
Governing Vessel, Conception Vessel, Yin Wei Mai, Yang Wei Mai, Yin Chiao Mai, Chong Mai. In this position the head is not held so far back that the Governing Vessel pathway to the head is totally closed.

YIN/YANG ORIENTATION
Yin In this exercise the legs are in a definite Yin formation and the arms are in a Yang formation. The spread palms with fingers turned away from each other unswitches the circular flow that would tend to keep the Qi in the Middle Tan Tien and allows the Qi of heaven to descend to the Lower Tan Tien. The feet spread to the sides on the other hand does retard the descent of the Qi of Heaven while encourages the ascent of the Qi of Earth. Actually the position is fairly balanced but tends to gather the Qi of Heaven and Earth in the Lower Tan Tien which is the residence of Jing which is considered Yin -Water-in comparison to the residence of Qi in the Middle Tan Tien which is considered Yang-Fire.

EXTERNAL/INTERNAL
External With the open palms encouraging the communication with Heaven and the leg position encouraging the communication with Earth this position creates a powerful exchange between man and nature.

ACUPUNCTURE POINTS
same as above

SPIRITUAL/ENERGETIC PROCESS
This position facilitates the mixing of Fire and Water Qi from inside the body and Heaven and Earth Qi from outside the body. The Microcosmic Circulation potential is not totally cut off by the head position. In Chinese Medicine the Knees relate to the Kidneys. The deep bending of the knees adds the potential of storing this Qi in the kidneys so that it can be used for health purposes and Spiritual Transformation.

On that subject, let me say that each exercise has an intended general effect. How much effect the practitioner gets depends, of course, on how correctly the exercise is performed and on the development of the practitioner. Different levels of development will modulate the exercises with different attributes. This is particularly true with standing exercises where with quiet mind, the Qi, is allowed to express itself as its innate intelligence dictates. The Kidneys are the storehouse of Qi. More Qi stored in the Kidneys allows that intelligence expanded options for expression.

COMMENTARY
This standing position is the most physically strenuous exercise in the Eighteen Buddha Hands QiGong system. That would be expected for a standing position following the chapter most associated with power building. The possibilities of balancing and collecting Qi from inside and outside the body are profound and the method ingenious.

CHAPTER THREE
THRUST FLOWERS TO LEFT AND RIGHT

The Three Flowers in Taoist QiGong relate to Jing ,Qi, and Shen. Jing resides in the Lower Tan Tien (Navel Charka)—Qi resides in the Middle Tan Tien (Heart Chakra)—Shen resides in the Upper Tan Tien (Brow Chakra).

Three Flowers meeting at the top is an expression relating to the point in cultivation where these three energetic substances have been refined, transformed, raised, and united at the top of the body (GV20—Crown Chakra) where the final work for enlightenment will occur. At this stage, all the Eight Extra-Ordinary Vessels are open and conducting refined Qi.

In Yoga and Esoteric Buddhism, the Threc Channels (Central Channel, Right Channel and Left Channel) must be opened and cleared to the Brow Chakra before the final work can begin in the Crown Chakra. In these cases, the Fire (PRANA) and Water (APANA) of the body must communicate and be acted on by Agni (Digestive Fire) to provide motive force for the transformations and clearing of the pathways. Next the Right and Left Channels (Ming Men Channels) must be cleared and activated. Various breathing techniques involving one nostril are often used for this process in Pranayama Practice.

In QiGong practices from many systems, exercises which feature one arm up and one arm down are said to strengthen the Spleen (digestive system). The usual explanation is that this position stretches the diaphragm in such a way that the digestive organs are massaged. This is mechanically true. At the same time this position pumps the Urinary Bladder Channels on the back and directly stimulates the Kidneys and Ming Men—whose upward channel underlies the inner Urinary Bladder Channel. The source of digestive fire is the Kidney Yang/Ming Men. This position causes the diaphragm to exert uneven pressure on the Lungs which results in the breath moving through one nostril more than the other.

Exercise One

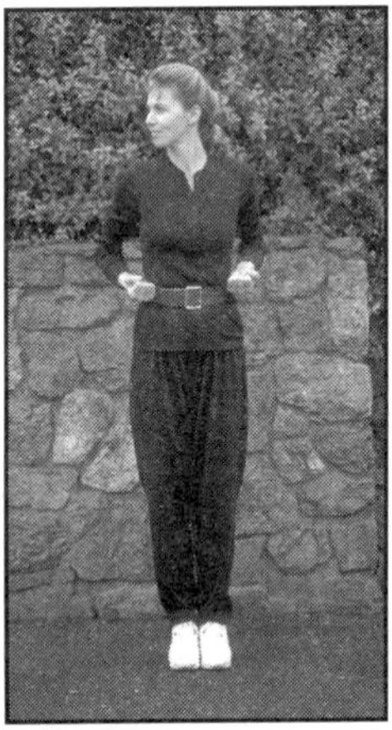

Three A

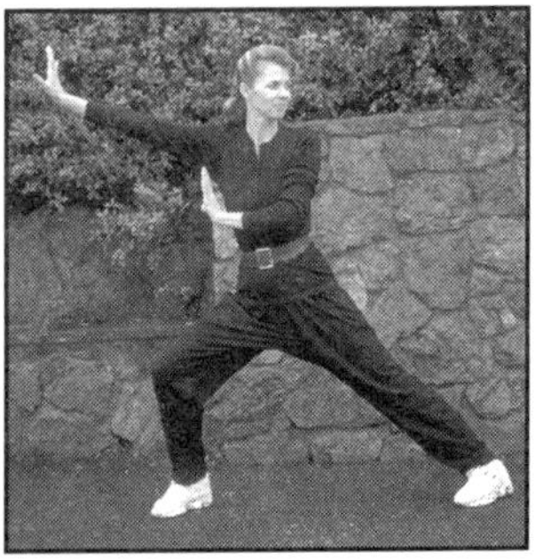

Three B

Stand with feet together fists at sides with palms facing upwards and look over the right shoulder inhaling to the Ming Men as in figure Three A.

With the right leg take a long step to the right while extending both palms to the right and exhaling to the Tan Tien as in figure Three B. During the step the head should turn 180 degrees so that you are now looking over your left shoulder with the left leg straight and the right leg bent.

Perform the revolving hands movement and return to the position shown in figure Three A.

Repeat this step out-exhale, step in-inhale sequence eight times.

Then perform the whole series in the opposite direction—stand looking over your left shoulder and inhaling to the Ming Men—step with the left leg to the left while pushing both palms to the left and looking over the right shoulder-exhaling to the Tan Tien—revolve hands and return to the standing position inhaling to the Ming Men.

At the end of eight repetitions of the above exercise you will be standing upright with fists at the waist looking over the left shoulder with your lungs full of air.

Look forward, exhale and breath normally.

BODY SYSTEMS
Respiratory System, Circulatory System, Digestive System, Genito-Urinary System

PRIMARY CHANNELS
All

EXTRA-ORDINARY VESSELS
All

YIN/YANG ORIENTATION
Balanced In this exercise the legs begin in a yang position and move to a Yin Position. The arms begin in a Yin position and end in a Yang position. The Qi inside the body moves up and down following the position of the hands. 'The overall effect is balance.

EXTERNAL/INTERNAL
External Both the Mind Regulation and open palm position facilitate communication with environmental Qi.

ACUPUNCTURE POINTS
LI4, SI3, P8, P7, P6, LU7, LU9, TB5, HE7, TB4, GV14, KI6, UB62, GV4, UB23, GB26, SP4, GB41, and Ki1 have all been explained in regards to the hand position before. GV14, meeting point of all the Yang Meridians, is strongly activated by turning the head as are GV4, Ming Men, and UB23 (the main Kidney point on the back). Ki6 and UB62, the Master Points of Yin Chiao Mai and Yang Chiao Mai respectively, are activated by having the

heel on the ground and foot raised during the stepping movement. GB41, Master Point of the Belt Channel and SP4, Master Point of the Chong Mai are activated by flexing the toes and foot upwards during the same movement. Kil is the point on the bottom of the foot that connects with the Qi from the environment. GB26, known as Girdle Vessel, is located at the level of the navel below the free end of the 11th rib. This point is activated by the position of the fist at the waist. The point is named for the Belt or Girdle Channel which it regulates. It also has a powerful effect on the Conception Vessel and Chong Mai.

SPIRITUAL/ENERGETIC PROCESS

As the exercise begins, Qi is inhaled to the Ming Men and the hands are drawn to the waist bringing Earth Qi upward to the Ming Men and Middle Tan Tien Qi down. As the body sinks onto one leg and the hands open , the exhale begins. Qi from the Lower Tan Tien is sunk to the Earth through the standing leg. The leg about to move becomes empty. The head turning at this point is already activating the storage and transformative functions of the Kidney/Ming Men and activating the Throat Chakra which links the sexual energy from the Lower Tan Tien to the Upper Tan Tien.

As the step is made and the arms extended the Qi is pushed out to the uppermost arm and the stepping leg. The arm connects with Yang Qi from the environment/sky and the foot connects with Yin Qi from the Earth. The head turning during this movement activates the Kidney/ Ming Men, the Throat Chakra, and the Belt Channel. On the return movement the foot being drawn in and the hands pulling in draw Qi from the environment into the body with an emphasis on collection in the Ming Men by the position of the hands and by inhaling back to the Ming Men.

The Qi inside the body follows the hands and moves from the Lower Tan Tien to the Upper Tan Tien and back, linking all three Tan Tiens and "Flowers".

COMMENTARY

While the Extra-Ordinary Vessels mentioned above are activated by this exercise, the main emphasis is on stimulating the transformative energies of Ming Men and its two Channels—the Left and Right Channels— and linking the Three Tan Tiens by the rising and falling of the Qi within the body

Exercise Two

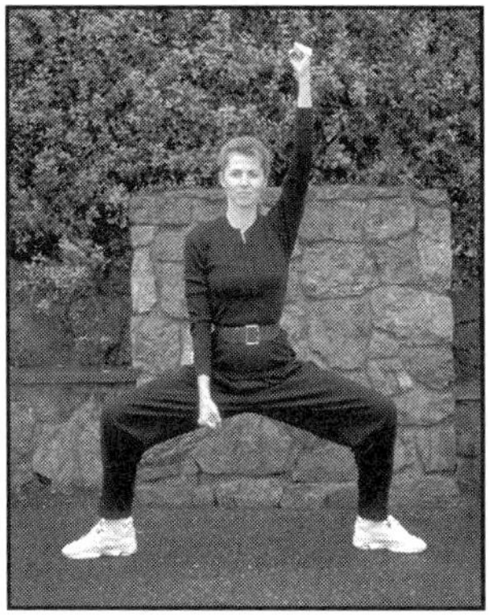

Three C

Spread the legs apart and bend the knees with the toes pointed out about 45 degrees. Raise the left fist above the head and lower the right fist straight down as in figure **Three C**.

Now change the arm positions, raising the right arm overhead and lowering the left arm downward.

Repeat this raising and lowering of the arms until each arm has been raised and lowered eight times while breathing normally.

BODY SYSTEMS
Respiratory System, Circulatory System, Digestive System, Genito-Urinary System

PRIMARY CHANNELS
All

EXTRA-ORDINARY VESSELS
In this exercise the strong up and down movements activate all the Extra-Ordinary Vessels. The feet are not spread so far apart that they restrict the Qi flows of Yang Chiao Mai and Yang Wei Mai.

The Yang Chiao and Yin Chiao Vessels actually form a circle from head to foot. The Yang Chiao which is associated with the Qi of Heaven flows down from the Head to the foot and the Yin Chiao which is associated with the Qi of Earth, flows upwards from foot to head. They meet in the Upper Tan Tien-Brow Chakra.

The Belt Channel is stimulated mechanically by the rise and fall of the waist (especially regarding GB26) and by the activation of Ming Men from the same movements. The movements and the activation of the Belt Channel affect the Governing Vessel, Conception Vessel, and Chong Mai. Yin and Yang Wei Mai are also mechanically stimulated.

YIN/YANG ORIENTATION

Balance The exercise features a Yin (but not extreme) leg position and rapidly changing arm positions which foster movement which is Yang.

EXTERNAL/INTERNAL

Internal The hands are closed to the outside and the feet are not in an extreme position so the Qi tends to move up and down within the body.

ACUPUNCTURE POINTS

This exercise depends on motion and the energy facilitating body position for its effects.

SPIRITUAL/ENERGETIC PROCESS

The most important function of this exercise is to stimulate the transformative functions of Ming Men —Agni or digestive fire. The moving up and down of the arms will facilitate communication between the Middle, Lower, and Upper Tan Tiens and activate the Extra-ordinary Vessels. Chong Mai, Conception Vessel, Governing Vessel, and the Belt Channel which will be especially affected due to the alternate stretching of the two Gall Bladder Channels.

COMMENTARY

As you can see from the above, this is a typical exercise that mechanically is good for the digestive system but has profound implications for more subtle transformative processes.

Exercise Three

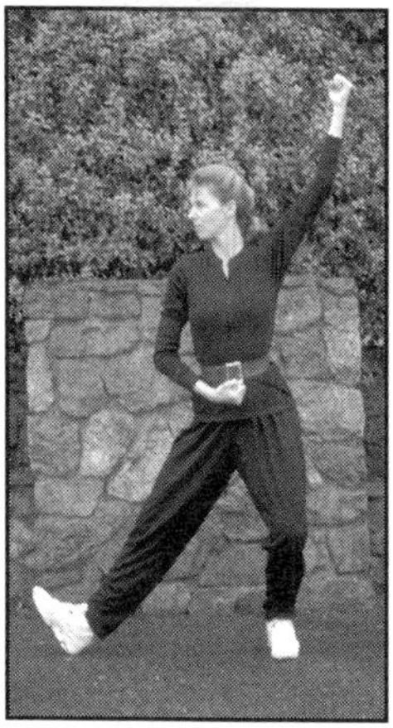

Three D

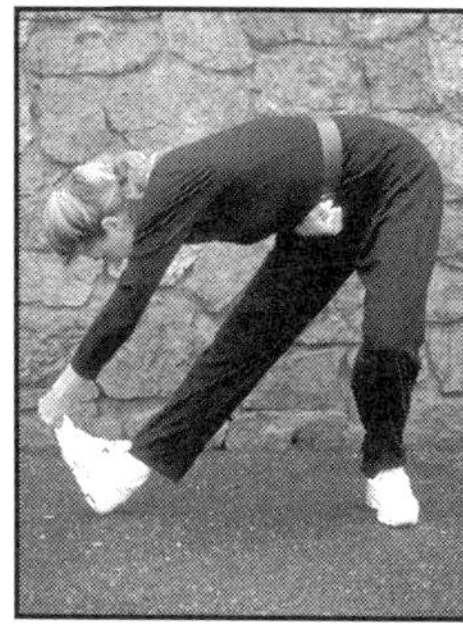

Three E

Assume the position pictured in figure **Three D**.

The left arm will be extended above the head, right leg extended resting on the heel, and right leg bent while supporting 90% of the body weight. The right fist will be held at the navel with the palm facing upwards and head turned to face the right side. Inhale to the chest as you assume this position.

Bend forward and touch the left fist to the right foot, exhaling to the Tan Tien as in figure **Three E.**

Return to the position shown in figure **Three D** while inhaling to the chest.

Repeat this bend down-exhale to the Tan Tien and raise up inhale to the chest movement eight times.

Repeat the sequence shown in figures **Three D** and **E** on the opposite side eight times.

When you finish this exercise, your right fist will be raised overhead with the weight of your body on the right leg and your lungs will be full of air.

BODY SYSTEMS
Respiratory System, Circulatory System, Digestive System, Genito-Urinary System

PRIMARY CHANNELS

All Holding the toes up is especially good for the Kidney, Liver, and Spleen while bending over and twisting are good for the Urinary Bladder and the Gall Bladder. The arm channels are not mechanically activated themselves but the up and down movement does indirectly affect them.

EXTRA-ORDINARY VESSELS

All Having the heel on the ground and the foot pulled up is the classic activator of the Yin and Yang Chiao Mai. Bending and twisting at the waist activates the Belt Channel. The bending also pumps the Conception and Governing Vessels. The up and down aspect tends to stimulate the Chong Mai and the Yin and Yang Wei Mais are mechanically stimulated. The Point section shows which Master Points are directly opened.

YIN/YANG ORIENTATION

Yang In this exercise, we have big movements which are somewhat balanced but only one foot is communicating with the Earth. The overall energetic emphasis is towards the top of the body with the bending actually facilitating the flow towards the top.

EXTERNAL/INTERNAL

Internal The hand is closed to the environment and one foot is disconnected from the Earth.

ACUPUNCTURE POINTS

UB23, GV4, KI6, UB62, SP4, GB41, CV6 see above CV6, point of access to the Lower Tan Tien, is activated by the placement of the hand below the navel.

SPIRITUAL/ENERGETIC PROCESS

The process in this exercise is the same as the previous one with one large difference. The bending motion in Exercise Three actually forces the transformed Qi to rise up the spinal cord and Min Men Channels, which makes this a very powerful tool indeed. The lower fist, representing the Fire of the Middle Tan Tien, is placed below the navel-Water of the Lower Tan Tien. The upper fist, which is also an extension of the Middle Tan Tien (Fire), is placed below the Lower Tan Tien (Water) at the foot bringing the Fire under Water in another way. The upstretched arm traveling to the foot very powerfully pumps the Ming Men Channel.

An interesting "twist" in this exercise is that the head stays relatively static while the body rotates beneath it, giving all the benefits previously mentioned regarding turning the head.

COMMENTARY
This exercise is the most powerful one in the system for mechanically leading transformed energy up the spine to the head.

Standing

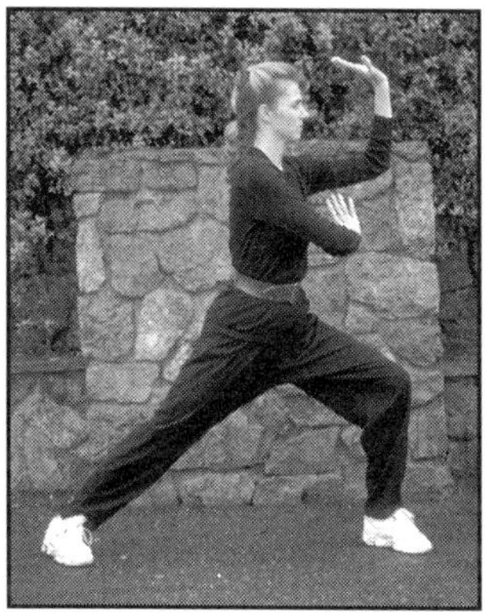

Three F

From the previous position exhale and move forward on your left leg until the right leg is straight and the left knee extends over the left toe as in figure **Three F**. At the same time move your right arm across your body until the fully flexed wrist positions the fingertips under the left armpit and extend the left elbow forward at shoulder level and bend the forearm upwards and flex the wrist backwards so that the palm faces up at the level of the head.

Hold this position for eight breaths.

Now reverse the previous position and hold for eight breaths on the other side.

This is the only chapter of the 18 Buddha Hands that has two standing positions following the exercises.

BODY SYSTEMS
Respiratory System, Circulatory System

PRIMARY CHANNELS
All

EXTRA-ORDINARY VESSELS
Governing Vessel, Conception Vessel Yin Wei Mai, Yang Wei Mai, Yin Chiao Mai, Yang Chiao Mai , Chong Mai, Belt Channel. These Vessels are activated by affecting their Master Points.

YIN/YANG ORIENTATION
Yang The overall emphasis of this position is to lead the Qi upwards on one side of the body.

EXTERNAL/INTERNAL
External The open palm encourages communication with the Qi from Heaven and the body position, through channeling the Qi to one side and up, encourages Qi from the Earth to be absorbed into the body.

ACUPUNCTURE POINTS
LI4, SI3, P6, P7, P8, LU7, LU9, TB4, TB5, HE7, SP4, GB41, KI6, UB62, P9, HE1—P9 on the lower hand is pointed towards and activates HE1 on the upper hand. HE1 is an important gateway for the Qi and Blood to circulate through the arm. This position of the hands helps to shift the energetic emphasis to one side of the body.

SPIRITUAL/ENERGETIC PROCESS
The straight back leg tends to collect Yin Qi from the Earth and the bent front leg helps draw the Qi up to the Lower Tan Tien. The hand position at the upper level draws the Qi upwards in the body with the lower hand directing the Qi to the opposite side of the body where the hand is raised. The end result is that all the transformed energy from the previous exercises in this chapter is channeled upwards and to one side to open one of the Ming Men Channels depending on which arm is raised.

COMMENTARY
This standing position is well suited to maximize the energetic emphasis of the three exercises in this chapter. The body is placed in the perfect position to allow the Qi to facilitate the opening, cleansing and transformational process stimulated by this chapter.

CHAPTER FOUR *OLD TREE STURDY ROOTS*

In the first exercise of this chapter, the stance is basically a one-legged stance but both soles are on the ground. This of course would increase the "rooting" of the body in the ground. The first exercise was probably the original so this explanation of the name is plausible. Another explanation, more interesting to me, is that the STURDY ROOTS refers to the Source Qi which is also called Root Qi by some authorities. An old tree takes a long time to grow and as my teacher says "has lots of time to gather the essence of the Sun and Moon" which would be transformed and stored as Root or Source Qi.

Exercise One

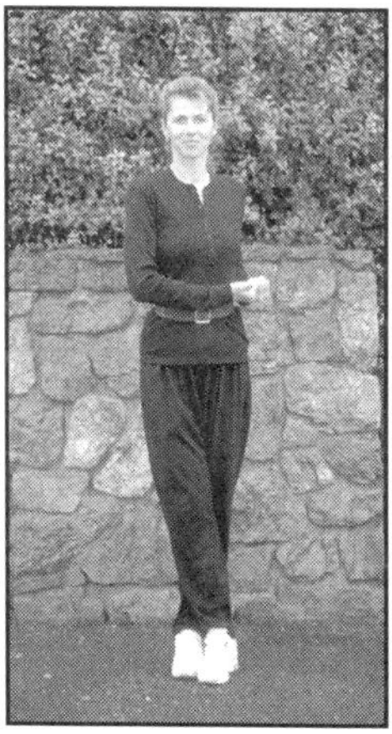

Four A

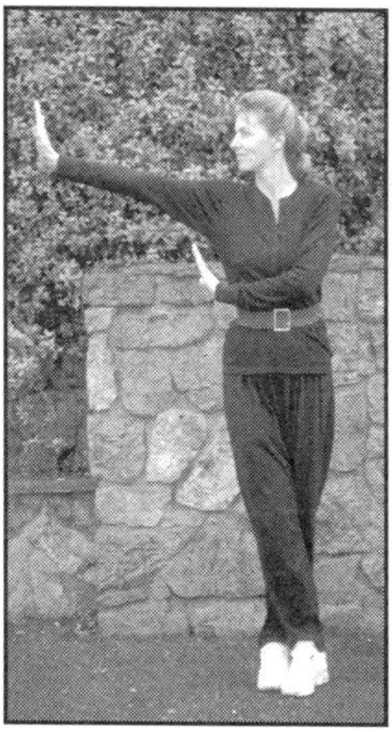

Four B

Place the left foot flat on the ground behind and to the right side of the right foot. Hold both fists level with the navel at the left side, with the palms facing, up while inhaling to the Ming Men as in figure **Four A**.

Extend both arms towards the right side with the fists turning into upright palms and the head turning to the right while exhaling to the Tan Tien as in figure **Four B**.

As the arms reach full extension perform the revolving hands movement and retract the arms to the position of figure **Four A** while inhaling to the Ming Men.

Repeat this extend-exhale and retract-inhale motion eight times.

When finished with the eighth repetition reverse the hand and foot positions and repeat the exercise on the left side for eight repetitions.

Return to standing with feet together and breath normally.

BODY SYSTEMS
Respiratory, Circulatory, Digestive, Genito-Urinary

PRIMARY CHANNELS
Lung, Large Intestine, Heart, Small Intestine, Pericardium, Triple Burner, Gall Bladder

EXTRA-ORDINARY VESSELS
All

YIN/YANG ORIENTATION
Yang The stance in this exercise is Yang. The movement takes place between the Lower Tan Tien and the Upper Tan Tien which promotes balance.

EXTERNAL/INTERNAL
External The open-palm revolving movement always opens the link between man and nature. The open palms crossing the Heart balance the Qi of the whole body, especially the Middle Tan Tien.

ACUPUNCTURE POINTS
LI4, SI3, P6, P7, P8, LU7, LU9, TB4, TB5, HE7. These points are activated by the turning of the hands. GV4,UB23 These points are activated by the turning of the waist. UB62, KI6, SP4, GB41 points are activated by the position of the feet. It is interesting to note in this position the GB41 points of both feet are placed together. GB41 is the Master Point of the Belt Channel. GB26 is activated by the position of the hands at the waist. GV14 is activated by the turning of the head and CV17 is activated by the lateral movement of the chest. CV6 is pumped by the breath.

SPIRITUAL/ENERGETIC PROCESS
After assuming the proper stance, the hands are raised to the waist inhaling to Ming Men which gathers some Yin Qi from the Earth via the weighted

leg and some Qi from the Upper Tan Tien to mix and activate the storage and transformative function of the Kidney/Ming Men. As the arms move outward with the exhale Qi is pushed into the ground through the weighted leg, out the palms to the environment, and up one Ming Men Channel to the Upper Tan Tien by the position of the arms.

The Belt Channel and Kidney/Ming Men are strongly activated by this movement as well as by the head turning to follow the upper hand. The head turning also activates the Throat Chakra. The hands claw and draw back to the waist bringing Qi from Earth via the weighted leg and Qi from the environment through the upper limbs. This movement also pumps the Ming Men Channel.

COMMENTARY

Somewhat reminiscent of exercises in the third section, this exercise pulls in Yin and Yang Qi to supplement the Source-Root-Qi while raising Qi from the Lower Tan Tien to the Upper Tan Tien. It accents the one-sided attributes of the Third Chapter more by hand and leg positions than by body movement.

ExerciseTwo

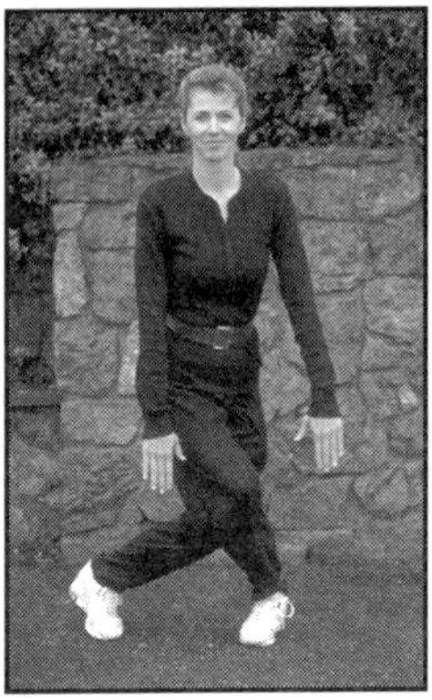

Four C

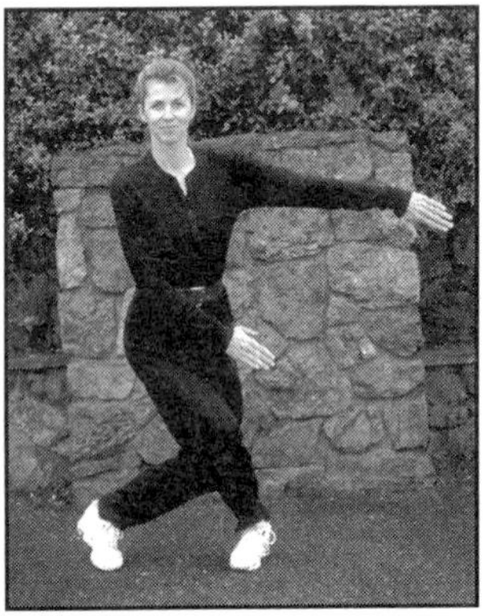

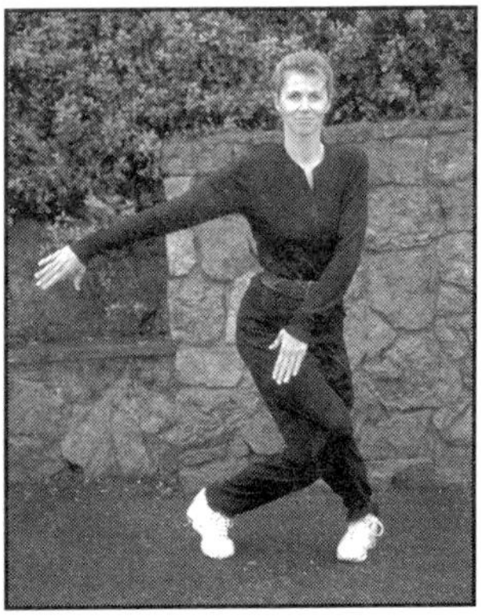

Four D

Move the left leg behind and to the side of the right leg with the knee of the left leg touching the mid-half of the right leg as in figure **Four C**. The right leg should support 90% of the body weight with the left toe just touching the ground. The arms should hang straight down with the palms facing the body.

Swing the hands to the left and right just under shoulder high as in figure **Four D** for a total of eight repetitions on each side while breathing normally.

Reverse the foot positions with the weight on the left leg and the right leg behind and to the left side of the left leg.

Repeat the arm swinging motion eight times to each side while breathing normally. Begin by swinging arms to the left and then to the right.

Stand with feet together and breath normally.

BODY SYSTEMS
Respiratory System, Circulatory System, Digestive System, Genito-Urinary System

PRIMARY CHANNELS
All

EXTRA-ORDINARY VESSELS
Yin Chiao Mai, Yang Chiao Mai, Chong Mai, Dai Mai—by foot positions and by movement the Belt Channel.

YIN/YANG ORIENTATION
Yin The main activity and movement are both confined to the Lower Tan Tien and below. The stance is low with Kil on both feet touching the ground.

EXTERNAL/INTERNAL
Internal Even though the palms are open they are directed at moving Qi inside the body.

ACUPUNCTURE POINTS
KI6, UB62, SP4, GB41 by foot position UB23, GV4 by movement.

SPIRITUAL/ENERGETIC PROCESS
Basically, this exercise takes the Yin and Yang Qi from the last exercise and mixes it in the Lower Tan Tien by the movement of the hands stimulating that function of Ming Men and by their position of Fire (palms as extensions of the Upper Tan Tien) being placed under Water (Lower Tan Tien). The body position and arm movements strongly activate the Belt Channel in its function of stimulating the "Moving Qi Between the Kidneys"

COMMENTARY
A simple but effective exercise to maximize the transformation of the Qi that is gathered in the previous exercise and prepared for the standing induced Qi flow to come.

This exercise very powerfully stimulates the "movement" aspect of the "Moving Qi between the Kidneys". If you look at the diagram of Ming Men (*see page 11*) you will see the lines linking the two aspects of Ming Men. There is a natural back and forth movement between the two aspects occurring along these lines.

If the two aspects represent the two Side Channels, this back and forth movement either constantly changes the polarity of the two (each of which is usually said to be of one polarity) or at least accents the energy in the channels alternately.

Supposedly when the Central Channel fully opens and is replete with transformed Qi both Side Channels will also be fully open and replete. In fact, the three Channels are said to merge into one. This merging could occur because the Channels actually enlarge due to their engorgement with Qi or perhaps the back and forth movement through the Lines of Ming Men becomes so rapid that practically they are one.

Probably both explanations apply. Even in one large column of Qi, the potential at different sides of the column could be different. Inner Vision could show one column with alternating emphasis on the opposite sides at one stage of development and three distinct channels that "feel" as one at another stage of development.

Direct experience through long years of training will give each individual his answer to that question.

Standing

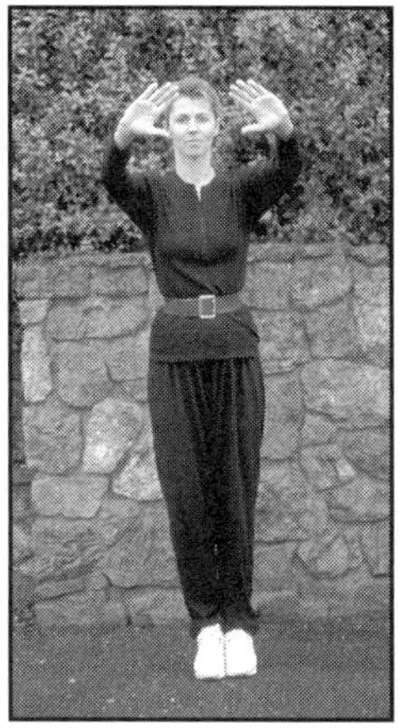

Four E

Stand as in figure **Four E** with the arms extended outward just above shoulder height and the palms facing forward.

Hold this position for eight breaths.

BODY SYSTEMS
Respiratoy, Circulatory, Digestive

PRIMARY CHANNELS
Lung, Large Intestine, Heart, Small Intestine, Pericardium, Tripel Burner

EXTRA-ORDINARY VESSELS
Governing Vessel, Conception Vessel, Yin Wei Mai, Yang Wei Mai—by hand position Chong Mai, Yin Chiao Mai—by foot position Yin Chiao Mai and Chong Mai by overall position encouraging flow to the Brow Chakra—Upper Tan Tien

YIN/YANG ORIENTATION
Yang The focus is on the upper Tan Tien

EXTERNAL/INTERNAL
Internal The palms are facing outward and able to draw energy from the outside as are the feet, but the purpose of this exercise in context is to move

the transformed Qi up inside the spine via Chong Mai and Up through Yin Chiao Mai. External absorption is secondary.

ACUPUNCTURE POINTS
LI4, SI3, P6, P7, P8, LU7, LU9, TB4, TB5, HE7, SP4, KI6, Yin Tang-Upper Tan Tein -Brow Chakra

SPIRITUAL/ENERGETIC PROCESS
This exercise simply puts the body in a position to induce the flow of the transformed Qi from the previous exercise to flow to the Upper Tan Tien while offering some potential to balance with nature.

COMMENTARY
This exercise allows the Transformed Qi to access the First Tan Tien, The three exercises in this chapter are a microcosm of the previous chapters with the addition of the Qi to the Upper Tan Tien, The chapter contains the gathering of Yang and Yin as the first and second chapters, the activation of the mixing, storing and transformative functions of the Kidney/Ming Men as the third chapter, and finally the rise to the Upper Tan Tien.

CHAPTER FIVE *NIGHT DEMON SEARCHING THE SEA*

Night is related to Yin and Demons are entities active at night. Night Demon refers to the focus of activity of this exercise being in the Yin region of the body.

The Sea refers to CV1 on the perineum, the lowest (Yin) point on the trunk. Searching means to bring attention to. At about the same time in the cultivation process that the Three Flowers Meet at the Top, the Five Qi return to the Source. In order for the Three Flowers to meet at the top all eight of the Extra-ordinary Vessels must be open and full of Qi. This state should cause the Five Internal Organs that store Essence to be full, whole and unblocked—directly communicating with their Source. Some sources link the Five Qi to the Five elements, which would still feature the Five Yin Organs as storehouses. In Yoga and Esoteric Buddhism, they are the Pranas and their associated spheres of influence—Ascending Prana, Descending Prana, Middle Moving Prana, Left Moving Prana, and Right Moving Prana. The Conception Vessel and Chong Mai meet the Governing Vessel in the Perineum. These three channels communicate directly with the Source. CV1 is the lowest point on the body (Yin) and GV20 is the highest (Yang).

The Three Flowers Meeting at the Top is a result of a Yang fullness and this must be balanced by Yin fullness at the bottom. One fullness must be supported and respond to the other. When the Three Flowers Meet at the Top certain signs will be apparent to the practitioner. A fully activated Sea Bottom will also produce noticeable signs. Thereafter when either area is activated the other will respond.

Exercise One

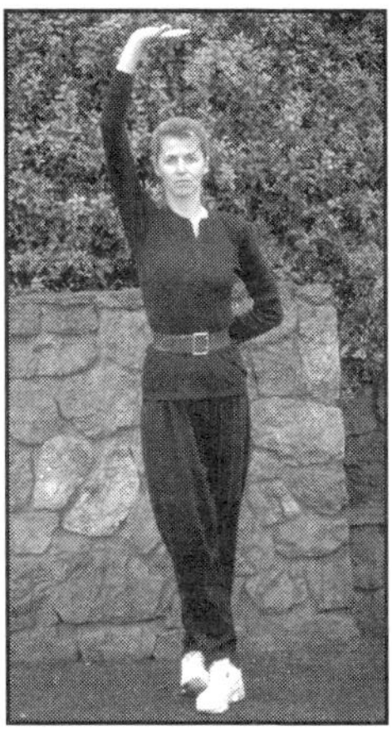

Five A

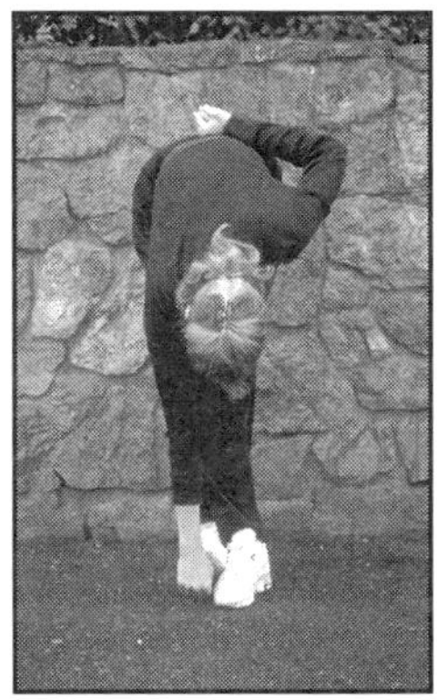

Five B

Move the left foot behind and to the right side of the right foot, resting the left foot on its heel beside the right heel and leaning the lateral side of the left foot on the lateral side of the right foot. Place the left arm, with the hand held in a fist, palm to the rear, behind the back parallel to the ground. Raise the right arm straight up from the shoulder with the palm facing upward while inhaling through the top of the head to the sky as in figure **Five A**.

Close the right palm to form a fist and bend forward while moving the fist down close to the body to touch the ground in front of the left foot and exhaling through the right foot and into the ground as in figure **Five B**.

Place the right arm, with the hand held in a fist palm to the rear, behind the back parallel to the ground and move the left hand from the back to just in front of the right foot with the palm facing upwards.

Straighten the body and raise the left palm close to the body from the feet to fully extended overhead while inhaling through the top of the head to the sky. Reverse the hand positions to return to **Five A**.

Repeat these bending over-exhaling straightening- inhaling sequence eight times.

At the end of the eighth repetition you will be standing with the left arm raised and the right arm behind your back. At this time reverse your feet, placing the right foot behind and to the left side of the left foot resting on its heel beside the left heel.

Repeat the exercise eight times on the left side and return to standing with the feet together breathing normally.

BODY SYSTEMS
Respiratory System, Circulatory System, Digestive System

PRIMARY CHANNELS
All

EXTRA-ORDINARY VESSELS
All

YIN/YANG ORIENTATION
Yang The stance is more Yang because only one sole touches the ground and the weight-bearing leg is straight. The arm movements are evenly matched up and down.

EXTERNAL/INTERNAL
External The open palms and stimulation of GV20 and KI1 create strong interaction with the environment.

ACUPUNCTURE POINTS
LI4, SI3, P6, P7, P8, LU7, LU9, TB4, TB5, HE7 by hand position GV4, UB23 by bending at the waist, CV1 by mind and any body regulation, KI6, UB62, GB41, SP4 by foot position , GV20 and KiL by mind regulation CV6 by breath TB4 and GV4 receive extra stimulation by the position of the fist at the back.

SPIRITUAL/ENERGETIC PROCESS

In the hand-up inhale position, the mind focuses on Qi moving through GV20 to the sky bringing transformed Qi to the Crown Chakra. During the inhale the Perineum, sea bottom, is raised slightly. As the fist moves down the body to the feet while exhaling, the Perineum is relaxed and the mind focuses on Qi sinking through Ki1 to the Earth. Ming Men is powerfully activated throughout by the position of the fist-TB4 Source Point of the Triple Warmer (Emissary of Source QI) on the back-GV4 (access point for Ming Men) as well as by the bending motion.

COMMENTARY

This exercise harmonizes man with Heaven and Earth. It also takes the practitioner out of the realm of the body (Lower Tan Tien-Jing and Middle Tan Tien-Qi) and into the realm of the Upper Tan Tien-Spirit. Jing and Chi can be manipulated through the body as they are in the realm of the physical, but Spirit transcends physical limitations. It cannot be manipulated but can be provided for.

Standing

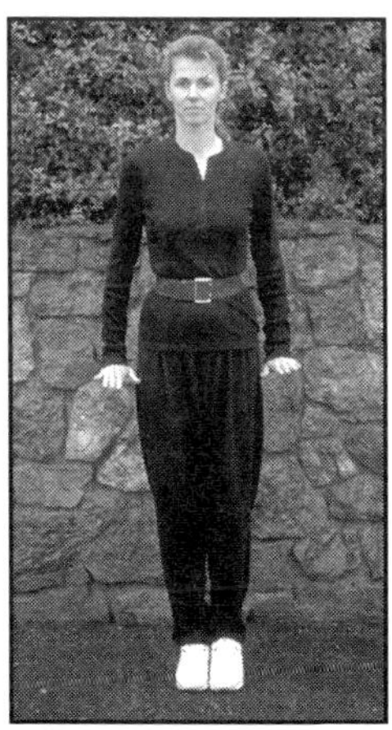

Five C

Stand with feet together arms straight down at sides with the palms held parallel to the ground as in figure **Five C** while breathing normally. Hold this position for eight breaths.

BODY SYSTEMS

All When the Qi is centered and replete all systems function efficiently.

PRIMARY CHANNELS
All
When the Qi is centered and replete all channels flow smoothly.

EXTRA-ORDINARY VESSELS
All When the Qi is centered and replete all Vessels flow smoothly. In this case the Chong Mai, Yin Chiao Mai, Governing Vessel, Conception Vessel, Yin Wei Mai and Yang Wei Mai are stimulated by action on their Master Points.

YIN/YANG ORIENTATION
Balance

EXTERNAL/INTERNAL
Balance The focus of this exercise is to center and balance the Qi of the body. In so doing, Qi from Heaven or Earth can be absorbed and turbid or excess Qi released naturally.

ACUPUNCTURE POINTS
LI4, SI3, P6, P7, P8, LU7, LU9, TB4, TB5, HE7, SP4, KI6. all by body position

SPIRITUAL/ENERGETIC PROCESS
Balanced centeredness. The body position and stance are Yang and the arm and hand position Yin. The hand position brings the Fire of the Middle Tan Tien below the Water of the Lower Tan Tien. This position allows the body to seek its own balance at whatever level of development is manifest in the practitioner.

CHAPTER SIX *FLASH PARRY OPEN WINDOW*

Flash Parry refers to turning the body to evade a sudden attack and Open Window refers to the physical pushing position used to open a large, heavy window.

Exercise One

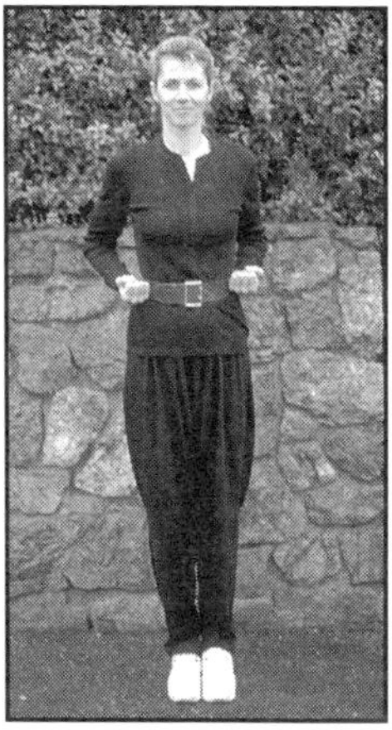

Six A

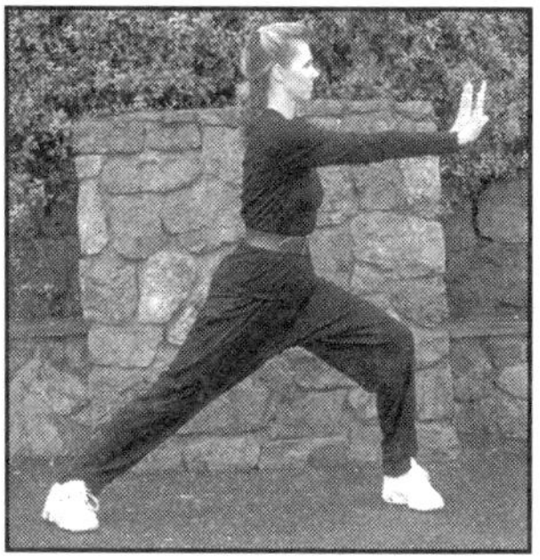

Six B

Stand with the feet together hands at sides. Raise the hands to the waist forming two fists with the palms facing upwards and inhaling to the Ming Men as in figure **Six A**.

Turn the right foot towards the right side and step to the right with the left foot, extending the right leg and bending the left leg while pushing both palms forward with fingertips pointing upwards and exhaling to the Tan Tien as in figure **Six B**.

Perform the revolving hands movement and step back with the left foot to the previous position while retracting your hands in fists to the waist and inhaling to the Ming Men as in figure **Six A**.

Repeat this step out-exhale step back to standing-inhale sequence eight times.

Perform the whole sequence to the opposite side eight times.

BODY SYSTEMS
Respiratory System, Circulatory System

EXTRA-ORDINARY VESSELS
ALL

YIN/YANG ORIENTATION
Balanced The legs move from a Yang to a Yin position and the arms move between the Lower and Upper Tan Tien. This is slightly in favor of Yang due to the big movement.

EXTERNAL/INTERNAL
External Absorption of external Qi is taking place from the hands and feet.

ACUPUNCTURE POINTS
LI4, SI3, P6, P7, P8, LU7, LU9, TB4, TB5, GV14, CV17, KI1GB26, GV4, CV6 all by body position and breath regulation as described earlier.

SPIRITUAL/ENERGETIC PROCESS
Raising the fists to the waist(GB26) while inhaling to Ming Men gathers Heaven and Earth Qi. Sinking, opening the hands, turning the foot on the heel, and beginning to exhale centers the Qi in the Lower Tan Tien and activates the Yin and Yang Chiao (Heel) channels and the Gall Bladder Channel which due to its intimate relationship with the Belt Channel activates that Channel and Ming Men. Stepping to the side and pushing while exhaling to the Lower Tan Tien pushes Qi out to the hands and feet to connect with external Qi. Collecting the hands and feet while inhaling to Ming Men gathers Yin and Yang external Qi.

COMMENTARY
This exercise provides a powerful method of gathering Qi from the environment to supplement the Qi of the body while moving Qi between the Lower Tan Tien and the Middle Tan Tien.

Standing

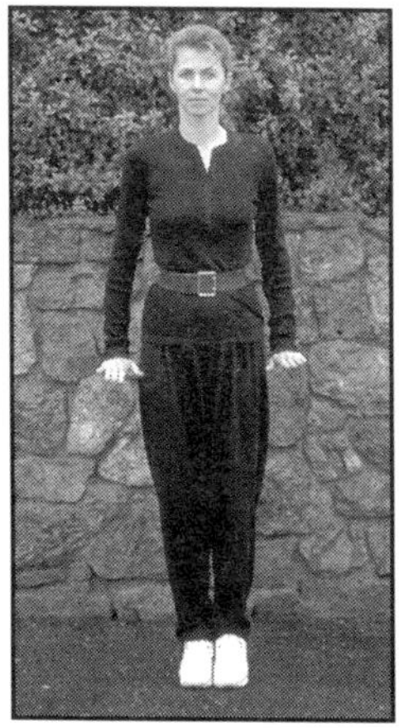

Six C

Stand with feet together arms straight down at sides with the palms parallel to the ground as in figure **Six C** while breathing normally. Hold this position for eight breaths.

see Chapter Five Explanations

CHAPTER SEVEN *WAI T'O PRESENTS STICK*

A stick can be looked at as a tool or opportunity. A presentation is made to a higher station. This exercise presents the opportunity to access a higher power—Heaven Qi.

Exercise One

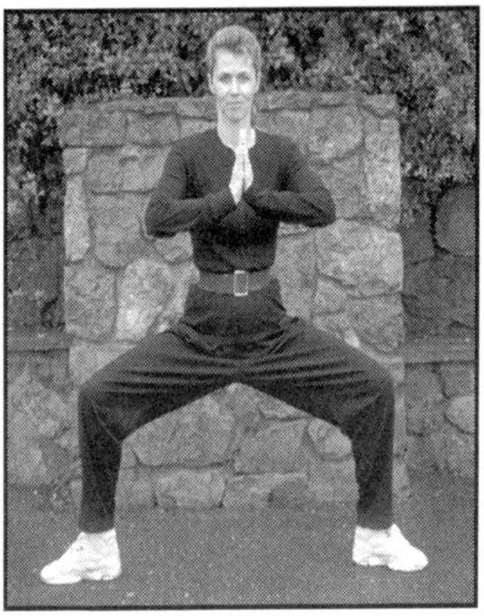

Seven A

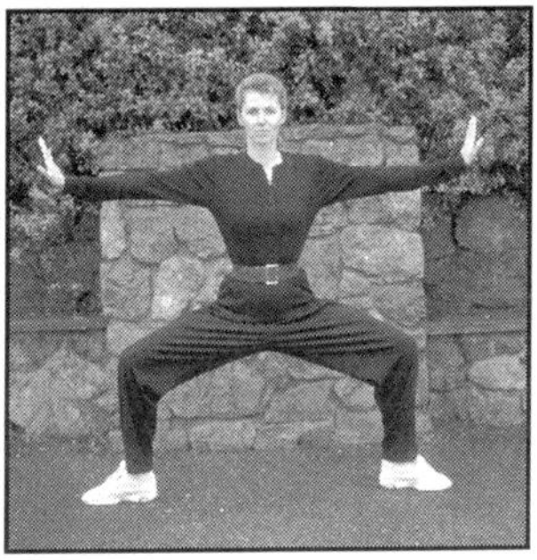

Seven B

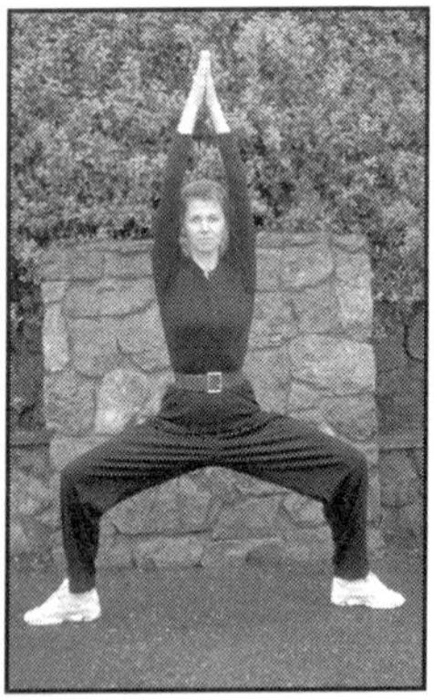

Seven C

Stand with the knees bent and legs spread apart with the palms touching in front of the chest as in figure **Seven A**.

Slowly spread the palms outward and to the sides inhaling to the chest as in figure **Seven B**.

Raise both palms until they touch directly over the head while exhaling to the Tan Tien as in figure **Seven C**.

Return both palms to the previous position while inhaling to the chest as in figure **Seven B**.

Bring both palms together in front of the chest exhaling to the Tan Tien as in figure **Seven A**.

Repeat this sequence eight times.

BODY SYSTEMS
Circulatory, Digestive, Respiratory

PRIMARY CHANNELS
All

EXTRA-ORDINARY VESSELS
All

YIN/YANG ORIENTATION
Balanced   The stance is Yin and the arm movements Yang.

EXTERNAL/INTERNAL
External   Absorption of external Qi takes place through the feet, hands and head (GV20)

ACUPUNCTURE POINTS
LI4, SI3, P6, P7, P8, LU7, LU9, TB4, TB5, HET, KI1, KI6, UB62, SP4, GB41, GV4. CV6 all by body position, breath and mind regulation.

SPIRITUAL/ENERGETIC PROCESS
The beginning position increases concentration and flow of Qi in the Middle Tan Tien, calms the Spirit and regulates the Heart. The leg position is not as extreme as in Exercise One of the Second Chapter so the Yang Channels (especially Yang Chiao Mai) are able to circulate Qi downwards more freely. Inhaling to the chest-Middle Tan Tien- and spreading open palms to the sides brings Yin Qi from Earth up and Qi from the environment in to meet in the Middle Tan Tien. As the hands are raised while exhaling to the Lower Tan Tien, mixed Qi from the chest is dropped to the Lower Tan Tien and Yang Qi from Heaven is absorbed into the Upper Tan Tien through GV20.

As the palms are lowered to the outstretched position while inhaling Yang Qi from Heaven pours down through GV20 to collect in the chest-Middle Tan Tien. As the hands return to the front while exhaling , the Qi collected in the Middle Tan Tien is pushed to the Lower Tan Tien for storage.

COMMENTARY

This is an advanced exercise to gather Qi from Heaven, Earth, and the environment (Mixed Yin and Yang). Mind regulation is the key—as usual.

Standing

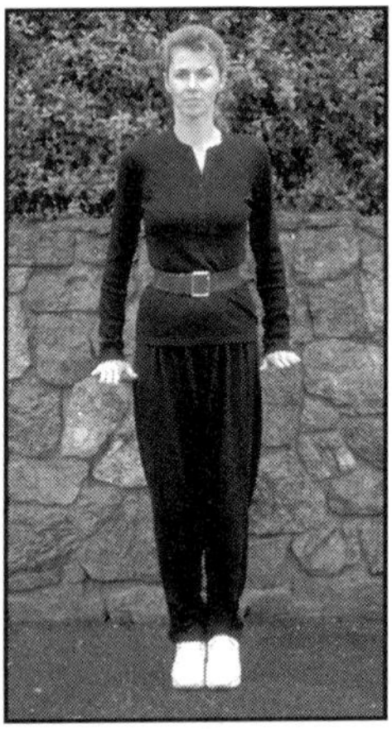

Seven D

Stand with feet together arms straight down at sides with the palms parallel to the ground as in figure **Seven D**. Hold this position for eight breaths.

see Chapter Five Explanations

CHAPTER EIGHT *OLD MONK MEDITATES*

The title of this chapter refers to one who has cultivated a long time. This cultivation results in the harmonizing of Heaven and Earth and Qi and Blood in man—essentially being "one" with the universe.

Exercise One

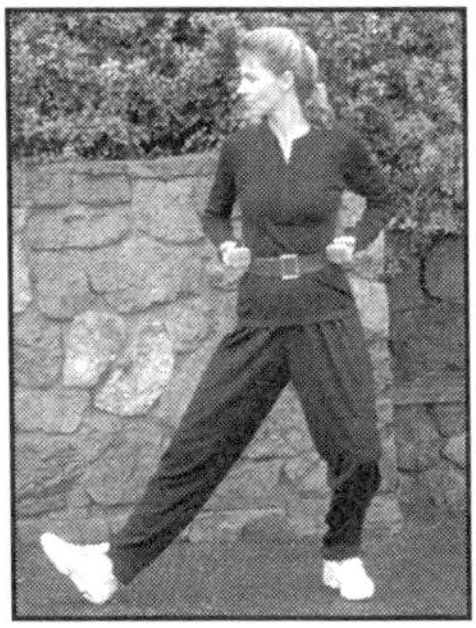

Eight A

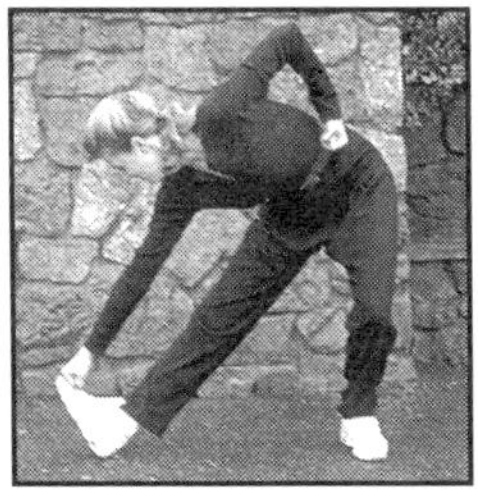

Eight B

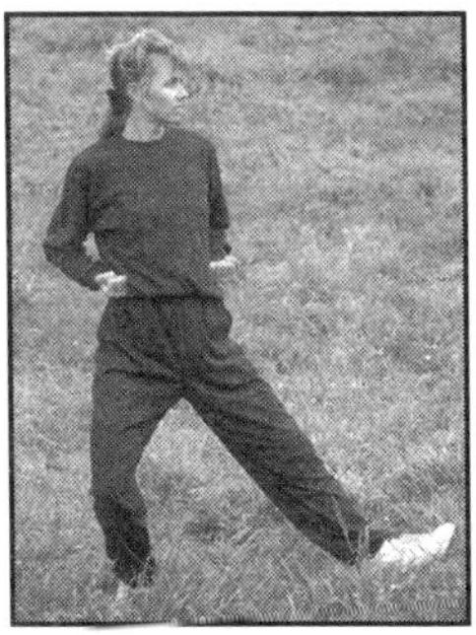

Eight C

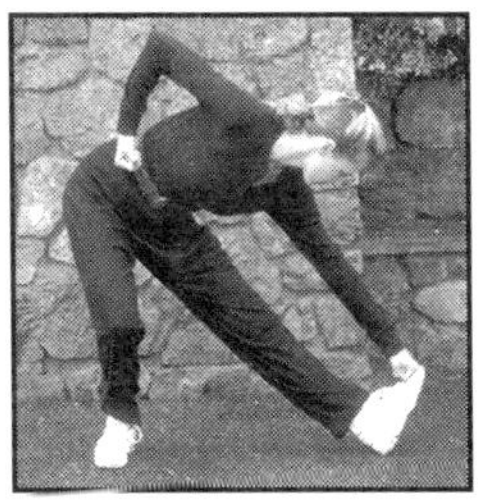

Eight D

Extend the right foot to the right side of the body resting on its heel with 90% of the body weight on the left leg. The left knee is bent. Place both hands in fists with palms facing up at the waist while inhaling to the Ming Men as in figure **Eight A**.

Bend at the waist and extend the right fist, with palm facing down, to the right toes while exhaling to the Tan Tien as in figure **Eight B**.

Return the right fist to the waist as you raise your body back up and change your stance so 90% of the body weight is on the right foot and the left foot is extended to the left side resting on its heel, inhaling to the Ming Men as in figure **Eight C**.

Bend at the waist and extend the left fist to the left toes exhaling to the Tan Tien as in figure **Eight D**.

Repeat this entire sequence of left and right movements eight times.

BODY SYSTEMS
Respiratory System, Circulatory System, Digestive System, and Genito-Urinary System

PRIMARY CHANNELS
All

EXTRA-ORDINARY VESSELS
Yin and Yang Chiao Mai, Chong Mai and The Belt Channel by the position of the feet stimulating the Master Points as well as the bending and pumping of the legs. Conception and Governing Vessels and Yin and Yang Wei Mai mechanically by the bending.

YIN/YANG ORIENTATION
Yin The stance is Yin and the hands do not raise above the waist.

EXTERNAL/INTERNAL
External and Internal Designed to bring Earth Qi to the Tan Tien and to circulate Qi in the legs.

ACUPUNCTURE POINTS
GV4 AND UB23 BY bending at the waist and GV4 and CV6 by breath. GB26 and SI3 by hand position.

SPIRITUAL/ENERGETIC PROCESS
Inhaling to Ming Men with fists at waist (GB26) stimulates the storage and transformational functions of Kidney/Ming Men. Exhaling from Lower Tan

Tien to leg as the fist travels down pushes Qi down to the foot especially through the Yang channels and Yang Chiao Mai. Inhaling as the fist is brought back to the waist and the stance is changed brings Qi from the Earth up to the Ming Men through the Yin channels especially Yin Chiao Mai and pumps the leg channels as well as the Kidney/Ming Men.

COMMENTARY
This is a truly industrial strength Qi of Earth gathering exercise. Keeping the hands in fists at the side is a technique to keep the Qi in the lower Tan Tien. The exercise not only gathers Qi from the Earth but also dramatically increases circulation in the legs.

Exercise Two

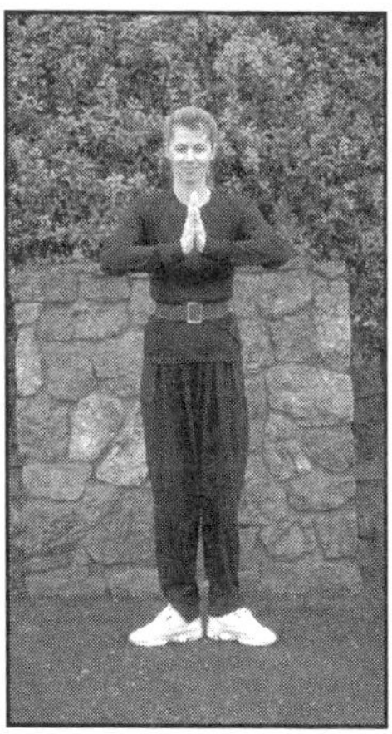

Eight E

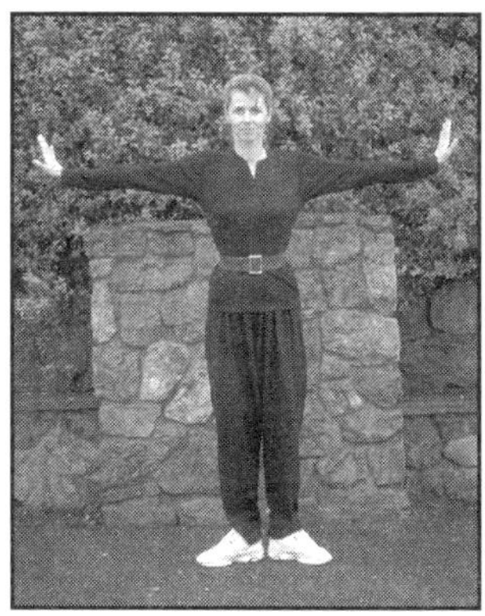

Eight F

Bring the heels of both feet together with the toes spread to the sides to form a toe-heel-heel-toe position. Hold the palms together in front of the chest as in figure **Eight E**.

Spread the palms outward and to the sides of the body while inhaling to the chest as in figure **Eight F**.

Return the palms to their previous position while exhaling to the Tan Tien as in figure **Eight E**.

Repeat this spread-inhale retract exhale sequence eight times.

BODY SYSTEMS
Respiratory System, Circulatory System

PRIMARY CHANNELS
Lung, Large Intestine, Heart Small intestine, Pericardium, Triple Heater

EXTRA-ORDINARY VESSELS
All The vessels with Master Points on the upper extremities are stimulated by the hand positions. The Vessels with Master Points on the lower extremities are passively opened by the leg position. Yang Chiao Mai is closed by the foot position.

YIN/YANG ORIENTATION
Yang Emphasis is on the upper body both in stance and in movement.

EXTERNAL/INTERNAL
External Designed to gather Yang Qi from Heaven, Yin Qi from earth and environmental Qi.

ACUPUNCTURE POINTS
SI3, LI4, P6, P7, P8, LU7, LU9, TB4, TB5, HE7 by hand position GV20 by mind regulation GV14, CV17 by arm movements CV6, GV4 by breath.

SPIRITUAL/ENERGETIC PROCESS
The beginning position with palms together increases concentration and flow of Qi in the Middle Tan Tien. As the hands spread to the sides inhaling Qi from Heaven, through GV20, and environmental Qi through P8 is absorbed into the Middle Tan Tien. As the palms return to the front while exhaling, the Qi in the Middle Tan Tien is transferred to the Lower Tan Tien for storage. The foot position allows Qi from earth to be drawn up and prevents Qi from heaven and environment from moving down through the legs via the closed Yang Chiao Mai.

COMMENTARY
Straight forward Yin and Yang Qi collection from outside the body by Mind Regulation and movement. The exercise also drastically increases circulation in the upper body.

Standing

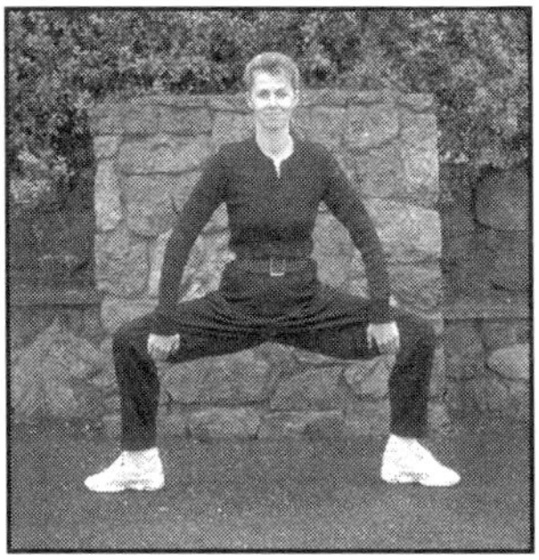

Eight G

Spread the legs and bend the knees while grasping the inner thighs just above the knees as in figure Eight G.

Hold this position for eight breaths.

BODY SYSTEMS
Circulatory System by stimulating SP10

PRIMARY CHANNELS
All

EXTRA-ORDINARY VESSELS
Yin, Chiao and Chong Mai

YIN/YANG ORIENTATION
Yin   The stance is yin and the arm position is Yin

EXTERNAL/INTERNAL
Internal   Position affects blood flow

ACUPUNCTURE POINTS
P8 and SP10 by hand position, KI6 and SP4 by foot position

SPIRITUAL/ENERGETIC PROCESS
Spleen 10-Sea of Blood- is one of the most influential acupoints that di-

rectly affect the blood. The balance and harmonization of Qi and Blood in the body is essential. True Qi, the mixture of post-natal and pre-natal Qi through which we normally function resides in the chest. P8 is the main point through which this Qi can be emitted for healing. This exercise allows the True Qi to directly harmonize with the blood creating a balance with and invigoration of the blood.

COMMENTARY
Simple yet profound energetic strategy for balancing Qi and Blood. In exercise one the circulation in the lower body was stimulated. In exercise two, the circulation in the upper body was stimulated. This standing posture harmonizes upper and lower circulations. The stimulation of P8 can invigorate blood and the cooling function of SP10 can purify the blood if necessary. Again we have the Fire from the Middle Tan Tien moved under the Water of the Lower Tan Tien with a special focus on the balance of blood and Qi.

In the overall chapter Heaven (Yang) and Earth (Yin) and Qi and Blood have been harmonized in man.

CHAPTER NINE *IRON COW PLOUGHS EARTH*

Ploughing the Earth is preparing Yin to bear fruit. Iron cow relates to an animal powerful enough to pull the plough and tough on the outside. This exercise stimulates and harmonizes internal and external Qi to promote energetic growth and Spiritual developement.

Exercise One

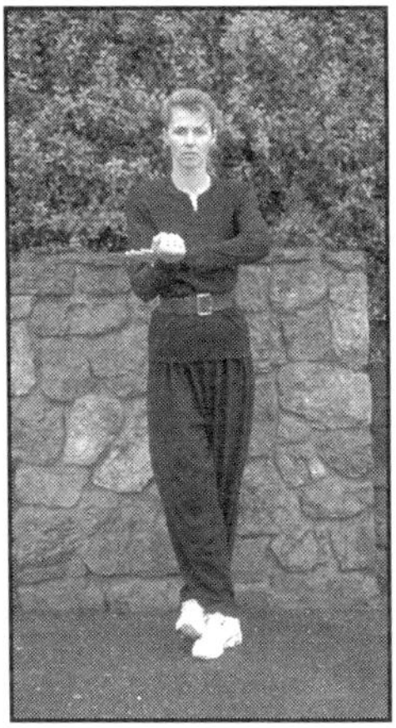

Nine A

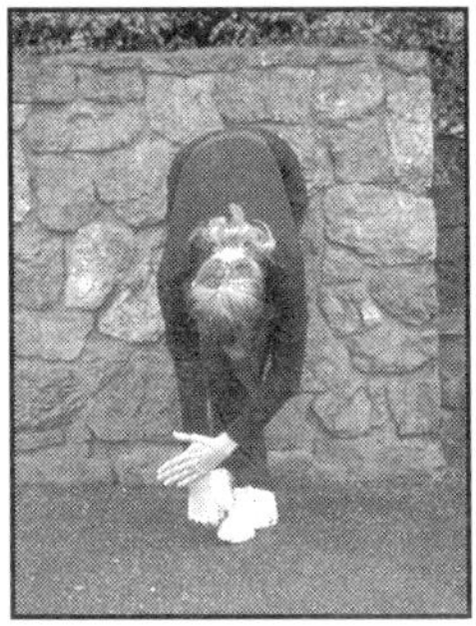

Nine B

Place the left foot behind and to the right side of the right foot. The left foot will rest on its heel beside the heel of the right foot and the left toes will lightly hook onto the top of the right foot.

Bend the right elbow and bring the right fist, with palm facing upwards, to a position approximately parallel to the ground. Vigorously slap the right forearm above the wrist with the left palm to halt its ascent. while inhaling to the Ming Men as in figure **Nine A**.

Bend forward extending the right fist to the ground and exhaling to the Tan Tien as in figure **Nine B**. Twist the right fist as you descend so the palm faces your body and the left palm rests on the back of the forearm above the wrist.

Return to the position in figure **Nine A** inhaling to the Ming Men and slapping the wrist.

Repeat this bend-exhale with straighten up-inhale eight times

Repeat the exercise on the other side for eight repetitions.

BODY SYSTEMS
Digestive System, Respiratory System, Circulatory System

PRIMARY CHANNELS
All

EXTRA-ORDINARY VESSELS
In many ways this exercise stimulates the flows of Qi in the Extra-Ordinary vessels more fully and powerfully than any other in the system. The bending motion affects the Governing Vessel, Conception Vessel, Belt Channel and Chong Mai. The foot position opens the Master Points of Yin and Yang Chiao Mai, Chong Mai and brings the two Master Points of the Belt Channel together. The slap on the wrist forcefully stimulates the Master Point of Yin Wei Mai (P6 Inner Pass), as does its proximity to P8 in the middle of the palm. As the low hand revolves downward P8 comes to rest on the Master Point of Yang Wei Mai (TB5 Outer Gate). The Yin and Yang Wei Mai control the Qi of the inner and outer aspects of the body as has been already mentioned. When the fist is at its lowest position, P6 and SP4 are in close proximity. These as you recall are the Master and coupled points of the pairing of Chong Mai and Yin Chiao Mai. LU7 and SI3 are stimulated by the turning of the wrist as the fist descends, activating the Conception and Governing Vessels.

YIN/YANG ORIENTATION
Yin The stance is Yang, but the focus of the exercise is at the level of the Lower Tan Tien and below.

EXTERNAL/INTERNAL
Internal The hands are held in fists throughout, closing off outside communication from P8. Only one foot touches the ground and there is some gathering of Qi from Earth, but the real ground being "Ploughed" is the Extra-Ordinary Vessel network, Ming Men, and the Lower Tan Tien.

ACUPUNCTURE POINTS
KI6, UB62, GB41, SP4, P6, TB5, SI3, LU7 as explained above. CV17 and Gv14 by the contraction and expansion of the chest during the bending. P8

by slapping. KI1 by weight and Mind Regulation, CV6 and GV4 by breath regulation, and GV4 and UB23 by bending motion

SPIRITUAL/ENERGETIC PROCESS
The breath regulation, bending and arm motions, and powerful activation of the Extra-Ordinary Vessels through their Master Points (while confining the activity to the Lower Tan Tien-Kidney/Ming Men) prepares (ploughs) the field(Lower Tan Tien) for explosive Spiritual/Energetic growth.

COMMENTARY
It would be hard to imagine a more powerful activation of the Extra-Ordinary Vessels in a simple exercise. The focus is kept in the Lower Tan Tien which represents the ploughed field awaiting the impetus to have life (Spiritual Development) spring upwards.

Standing

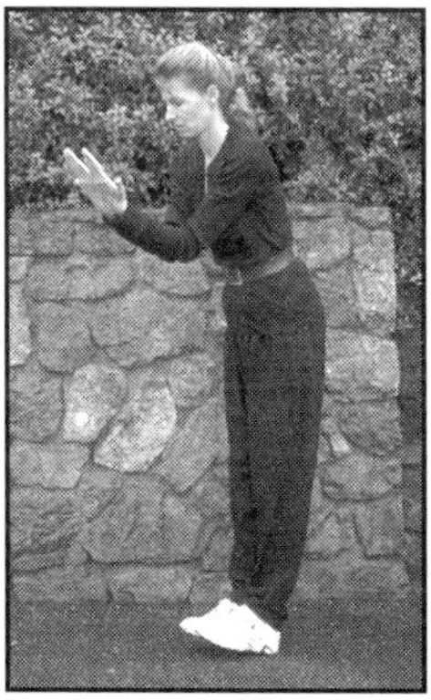

Nine C

Stand with feet together, toes lifted, and weight on the heels while looking into the palms as in figure **Nine C**.

Hold this position for eight breaths.

BODY SYSTEMS
Circulatory, Respiratory

PRIMARY CHANNELS

All This position of the arms is used in some styles of QiGong to affect the Liver, which is in charge of the free flow of Qi throughout the body and storage of blood, among other things.

EXTRA-ORDINARY VESSELS

Yin and Yang Chiao Mai, Chong Mai, and the Belt Channel by foot position, Governing Vessel and Conception Vessel by the proximity of both sets of Master Points in the hand position.

YIN/YANG ORIENTATION

Yang The entire emphasis of this position is upwards movement. Even the feet are both uplifted.

EXTERNAL/INTERNAL

Internal The hands are open but direct Qi to the Upper Tan Tien and Kil is lifted off the ground on both feet. Even the head is bent slightly forward minimizing the link between GV20 and Heaven.

ACUPUNCTURE POINTS

KIL, UB62, SP4, GB41, SI3, LU7 as stated above Yin Tang (Upper Tan Tien) and P8 by mind regulation and of course spreading the palm for P8. Lung 9 by the two points being in close proximity. GV14 by the spread back UB23 and GV4 by waist position.

SPIRITUAL/ENERGETIC PROCESS

The body position alone promotes the flow of Qi upwards to the First Tan Tien. With the addition of Mind Regulation emitting Qi from P8 to Yin Tan (Upper Tan Tien), we have the most powerful Brow Chakra energizer in the System.

COMMENTARY

After gathering Qi in the Lower Tan Tien, activating the transformative function of the Ming Men and powerfully opening the whole Extra-Ordinary Vessel network in the previous exercise, this position offers a profound energetic opportunity to manifest refined Qi at the level of the Upper Tan Tien—Brow Chakra.

CHAPTER TEN *GREEN DRAGON WAGS ITS TAIL*

Green Dragon refers to the wood element whose energetic nature is explosive upward growth. Wagging the tail refers to the sweeping arm movements.

Exercise One

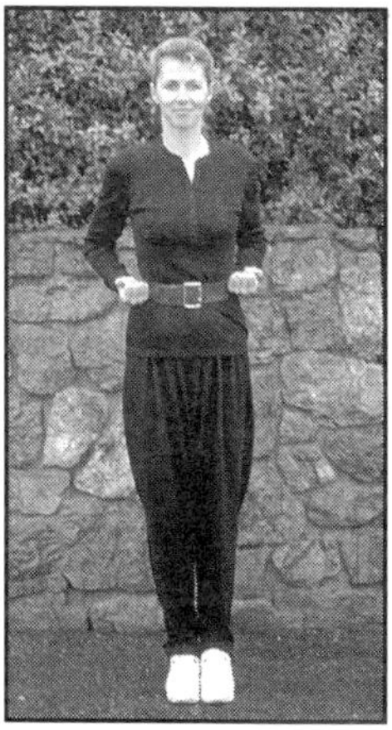

Ten A

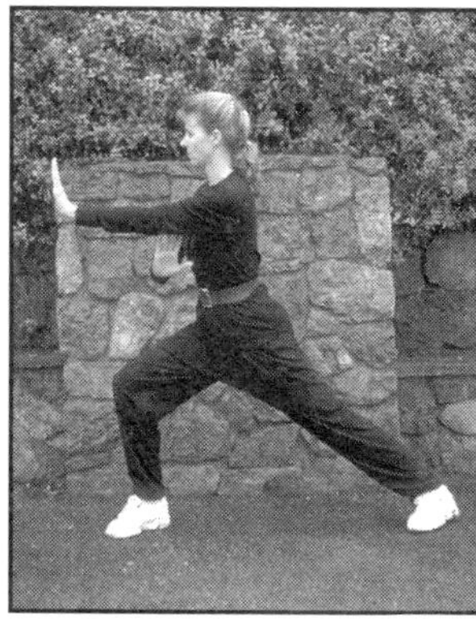

Ten B

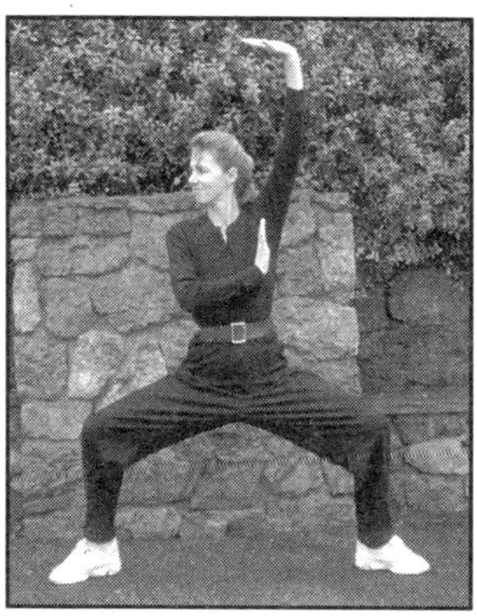

Ten C

Stand with the feet together. Raise the hands in fists to the waist while inhaling to the Ming Men as in figure **Ten A**.

Step to the right with the right leg, extending the left leg and bending the right leg. As you step, extend the left palm forward at shoulder level and push the right palm across the body with the right fingertips pointing at the left armpit, exhaling to the Tan Tien as in figure **Ten B**.

Twist the body to the left making a wide circle with the left hand from the extended forward position down and to the raised overhead position shown in figure **Ten C** as you inhale to the Ming Men.

Return to the position shown in Ten A while holding the breath.

Repeat this step out-exhale twist the body-inhale sequence eight times.

Repeat the same exercise on the other side for eight repetitions.

BODY SYSTEMS
Circulatory System, Respiratory System, Digestive System, Genito-Urinary System

PRIMARY CHANNELS
All

EXTRA-ORDINARY VESSELS
All By stimulation of their Master Points in the hand and foot movements and positions.

YIN/YANG ORIENTATION
Yang The Legs are in Yin and Yang positions but this is mediated by their movement-Yang. The arms move in both Yin and Yang directions but the focus is upward-Yang.

EXTERNAL/INTERNAL
Internal Although the palms are exposed the focus of this exercise is movement of Qi within the body. There is some interaction with the environment but it is mainly harmonizing in nature.

ACUPUNCTURE POINTS
LI4, SI3, P6, P7, P8, TB4, TB5, LU7, LU9, HE7, CV6, GV4, UB23, GV14, CV17, GB41, SP4, Ki6, UB62, HE1, GV20

SPIRITUAL/ENERGETIC PROCESS

Raising the fists to the level of the Lower Tan Tien at the beginning while inhaling concentrates the Qi in the Lower Tan Tien. Stepping out, opening fists exhaling and pushing the arm out sinks the Qi back to the Earth through the weighted leg and then pushes Qi from the Earth to the extremities. Sweeping the hand down the front and circling it to overhead first concentrates Qi in the Lower Tan tien then vigorously pulls it to the top. The movement and position of the less active hand directs the Qi to one side of the body thereby focusing the exercise of thrusting Qi up either the right or left Channel—Ming Men.

COMMENTARY

This exercise is extremely powerful in opening and clearing the left and right channels—Ming Men. It is different from earlier exercises for that purpose in that it not only pumps but also packs. In other words, a large portion of the Qi that is thrust upwards stays in the channel on the recovery movement of dropping the hand to the side to push again so throughout the exercise the channel is being packed with Qi. Another interesting point concerning this exercise is the movement of the body under the head. We already know that moving the head from side to side activates the storage and transformational functions of the Kidney/Ming Men and the Belt Channel. In this exercise the body moves powerfully under the head creating the same result and of course stimulating the throat chakra, which links the Lower Tan Tien with the Upper Tan Tien.

Exercise Two

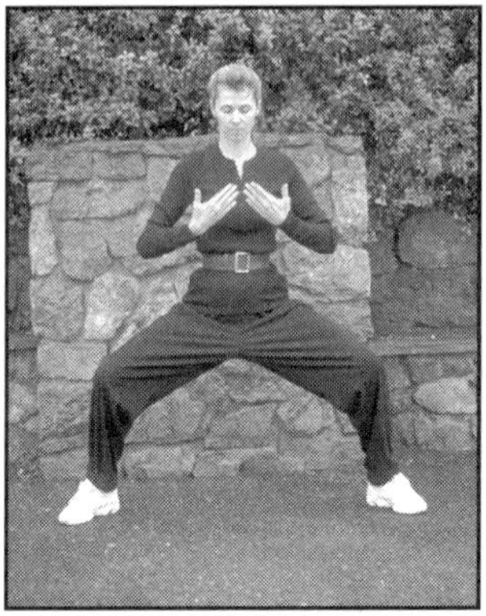

Ten D

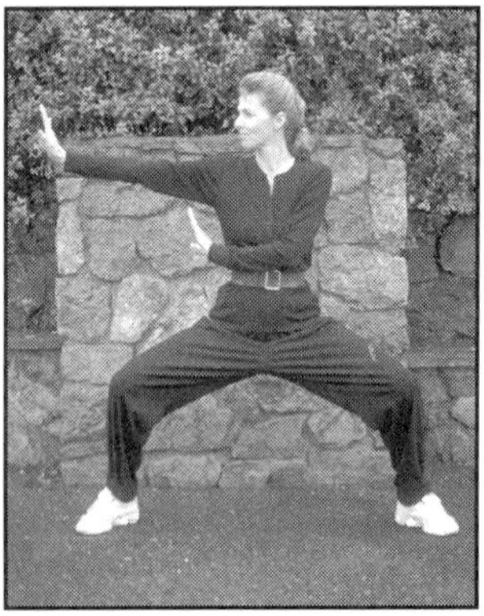

Ten E

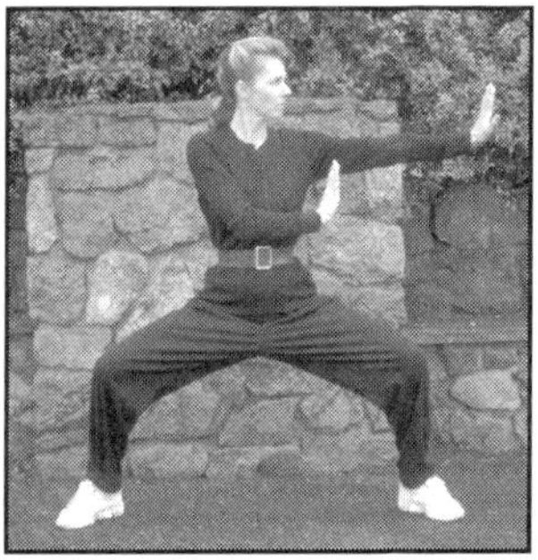

Ten F

Spread the legs and bend the knees as in figure **Ten D** while inhaling to the Ming Men and raising palms to chest.

Push both palms to the right side with vigor while exhaling to the Tan Tien as in figure **Ten E**.

Retract the hands with the palms facing the chest while inhaling to the Ming Men.

Push both palms to the left side with vigor while exhaling to the Tan Tien as in figure **Ten F**.

Retract the hands with the palms facing the chest while inhaling to the Ming Men.

Repeat this left/right sequence eight times.

BODY SYSTEMS
All

PRIMARY CHANNELS
All

EXTRA-ORDINARY VESSELS
All

YIN/YANG ORIENTATION
Balanced The stance is Yin and the arms remain at the Middle Tan Tien level. The movement is neither up nor down but is movement, a Yang attribute, to balance the Yin stance.

EXTERNAL/INTERNAL
External The open palms connect man with nature via P8.

ACUPUNCTURE POINTS
Same as above

SPIRITUAL/ENERGETIC PROCESS
As the palms raise to the chest during the inhale, Qi from the lower Tan Tien is drawn to the Middle Tan Tien. As the open palms are vigorously thrust to the sides, the exhale is focused on the Lower Tan Tien. Qi sinks to the Lower Tan Tien and is pushed to the extremities. The hands are then drawn into the mid chest inhaling. When P8 passes CV17 the Qi of the entire body is balanced and the Heart is harmonized. The vigorous thrusting of the palms outward allows excess Qi to be expelled to the environment relieving any potential problems of excess Qi buildup from the previous exercise.
GV20 may be activated by Mind Regulation.

COMMENTARY
This exercise is really a safety valve for the previous one. In the first exercise large amounts of Qi were packed into the upper body. This can be stressful if the practitioner is not developed enough to naturally harmonize the excess Qi. The stress will be felt by the Heart. This exercise allow excess Qi to be emitted and the Heart to be harmonized.

Standing

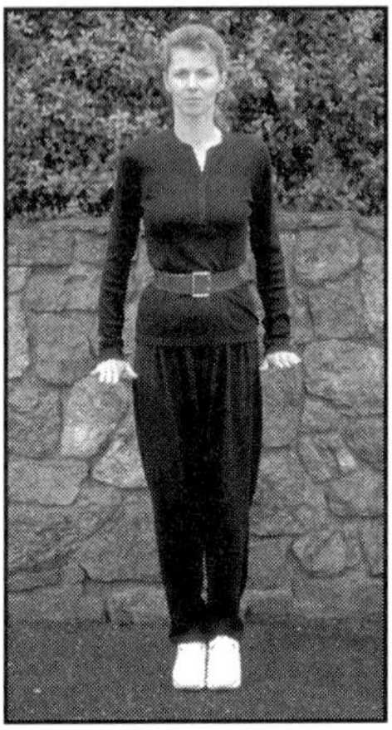

Ten G

Stand with feet together hands at the sides with palms parallel to the ground as in figure **Ten G** while breathing normally.

Hold this position for eight breaths.

see Chapter Five Explanations

CHAPTER ELEVEN *VAULT A HORSE LEFT AND RIGHT*

The name of this chapter reflects the physical movement of the first exercise.

Exercise One

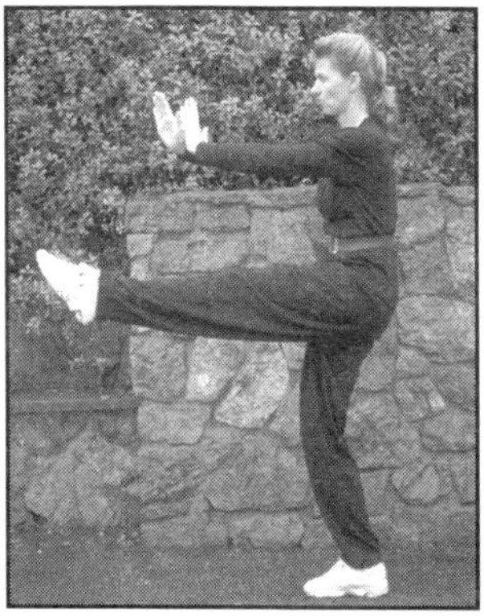

Eleven A

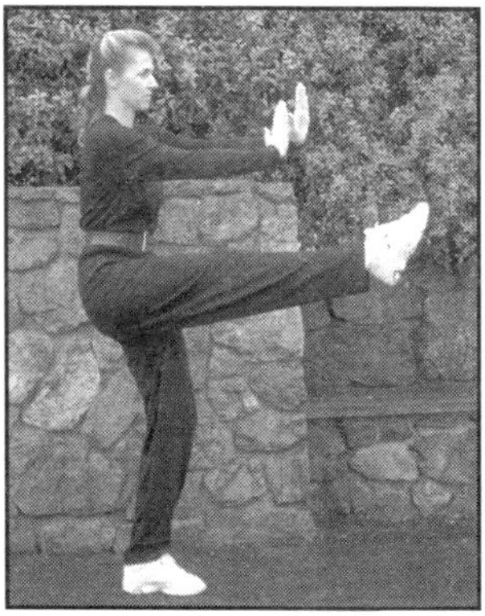

Eleven B

From a standing position turn to the right and extend the right arm, with the fingers of the open palm pointing upward, to the right side. At the same time extend the left leg and the left palm, with fingers pointing upward, outward to the right side while exhaling to the Tan Tien. The left palm should contact the right wrist with force as in figure **Eleven A**.

Return to the standing position facing forward while inhaling to the Ming Men.

Repeat this sequence to the left side as in figure **Eleven B**.

Do eight repetitions of this left-right movement ending facing forward in the standing position.

BODY SYSTEMS
Circulatory System, Digestive System, Respiratory System, Genito-Urinary System

PRIMARY CHANNELS
All

EXTRA-ORDINARY VESSELS
All

YIN/ YANG ORIENTATION
Yang The stance is moving and often on one foot only. The arm movements are vigorous and emphasize rising, both Yang traits.

EXTERNAL/INTERNAL
Internal Despite the open palms there is no major Qi exchange with the environment. Ki1 is often not in contact with the ground.

ACUPUNCTURE POINTS AFFECTED—LI4, SI3, P6, P7, P8, LU7, LU9, TB4, TB5, HE7 by hand position UB62 ,Ki1, SP4, GB41 By foot position CV17, GV14 by expansion and contraction of the chest, GV4, CV6 by breath regulation UB23, GC4 by waist bending.

SPIRITUAL/ENERGETIC PROCESS
As the inhale is directed to the Ming Men/Kidney, Qi is gathered in the Lower Tan Tien. Exhaling to CV6 while raising the leg and forcefully joining the upper limbs moves Qi from the Lower Tan Tien to the extremities and gathers Qi in the limbs. Inhaling to Ming Men while returning to the upright position gathers the mobilized Qi back to the Kidney/ Ming Men. The turning, bending and limb movements all strongly activate the transformational and storage functions of the Kidney/Ming Men. Turning especially activates the Gall Bladder which in turn stimulates the Belt Channel. The Belt channel focuses even more activity on the "Moving Qi Between the Kidneys".

COMMENTARY
This is another exercise that gathers large amounts of Qi in the Lower Tan Tien for storage and transformation. Leaving the palm open in the slapping motion allows any excess Qi generated to emit to the environment rather than put too much stress on the Heart. Basically the Lower Tan Tien is considered Yin compared to the Middle Tan Tien so we have a large amount of Yang activity generating Yin—developing the Yin in Yang. The exercise also powerfully increases Qi circulation in the extremities.

Exercise Two

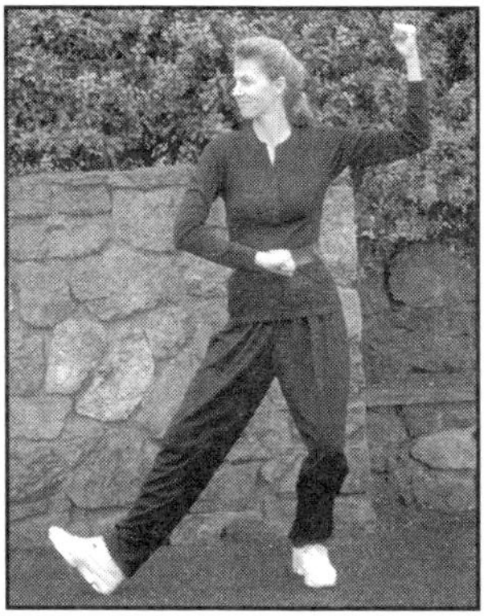

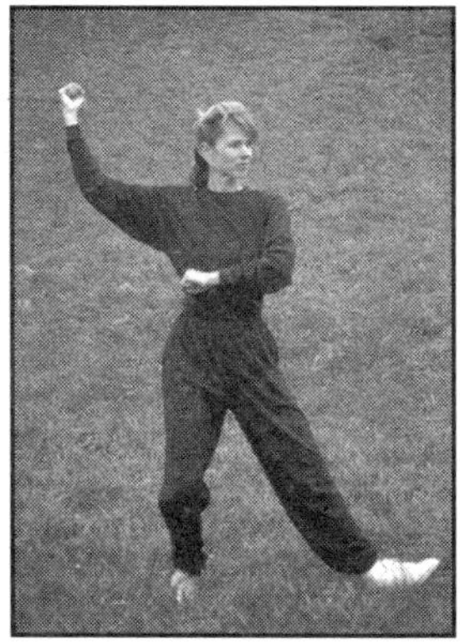

Eleven C *Eleven D*

Extend the right leg out to the right side of the body resting on its heel. Raise the left hand in a fist slightly overhead and place the right fist at side level with navel while inhaling to the Tan Tien as in figure **Eleven C**.

Turn to the other side reversing the foot and hand positions. Move the top hand down and the bottom hand up the midline of the body. Exhale to the Tan Tien until the hands cross and then inhale to the Ming Men as in figure **Eleven D**.

Perform this right-left sequence eight times.

BODY SYSTEMS
Respiratory System, Circulatory System, Digestive System, Genito-Urinary System

PRIMARY CHANNELS
All

EXTRA-ORDINARY VESSELS
Yin and Yang Chiao Mai, Chong Mai and Belt Channel by foot positions. The up and down motion of the hands stimulates Conception Vessel as it

takes place in line with and close to the Channel. Up and down motion always tends to stimulate the Conception and Governing Vessels and Chong Mai.

YIN/YANG ORIENTATION
Yin The stance is Yin (modulate by the toe up movement) and the arm movements are not large nor extended above the head. Even though the focus of this exercise is to move Qi up and down, the overall construction of the form is Yin. Here we have a case of exercising the Yang in Yin.

EXTERNAL/INTERNAL
Internal The hands remaining "closed" and the constant raising of Ki1 on one leg keeps the focus of this exercise internal, although there is some interaction with the Earth.

ACUPUNCTURE POINTS
UB62, KIL, SP4, GB41 by foot position CV6 and GV4 by breath GV4 and UB23 by side to side waist and arm raising motion CV17 by fists crossing close and GV14 BY alternate arm raising.

SPIRITUAL/ENERGETIC PROCESS
We begin the exercise with a large amount of concentrated Qi being stored and transformed in the Lower Tan Tien . As we inhale and raise the fist that Qi is moved subtly but powerfully up the Right or Left Side Channel— Ming Men— to the head, The lower fist keeps the Qi channeled to one side of the body or the other. The fist moving to center as the body starts to descend concentrates the Qi in the Upper Tan Tien-Brow Chakra- before descending down the Conception Vessel .

COMMENTARY
Both exercises in this chapter are high level and quite subtle. Dealing with the Yin in Yang and the Yang in Yin is a delicate and a very profound experience.

Standing

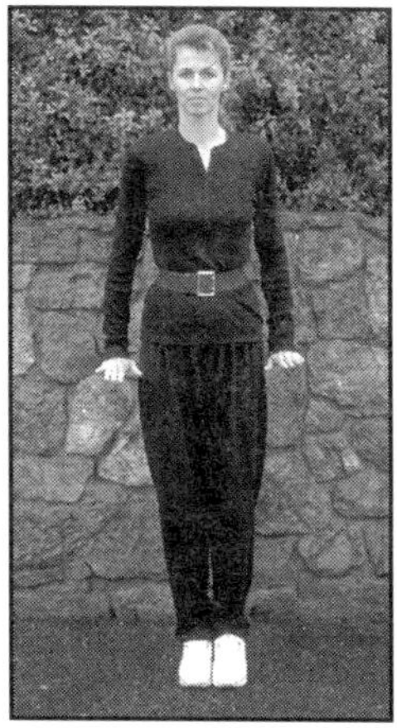

Eleven E

Stand with feet together hands at the sides with the palms parallel to the ground as in figure Eleven E. Hold this position for eight breaths.

.

see Chapter Five Explanations

CHAPTER TWELVE *SWALLOW FLINGS WATER*

When Swallows gather water from a lake or stream, they swoop down and rise up in smooth motions. This chapter is named for the swooping nature of the motions.

Exercise One

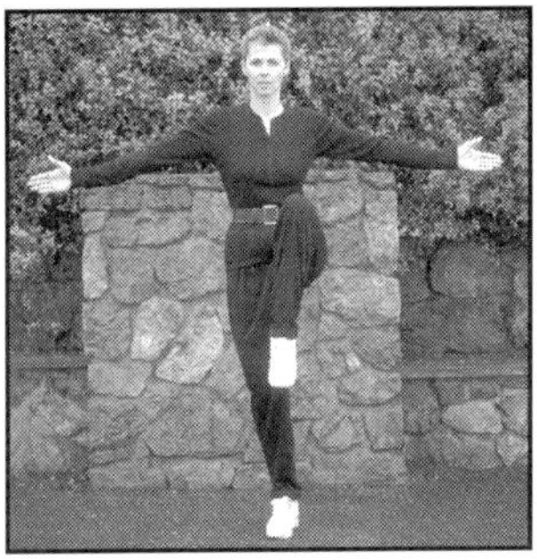

Twelve A

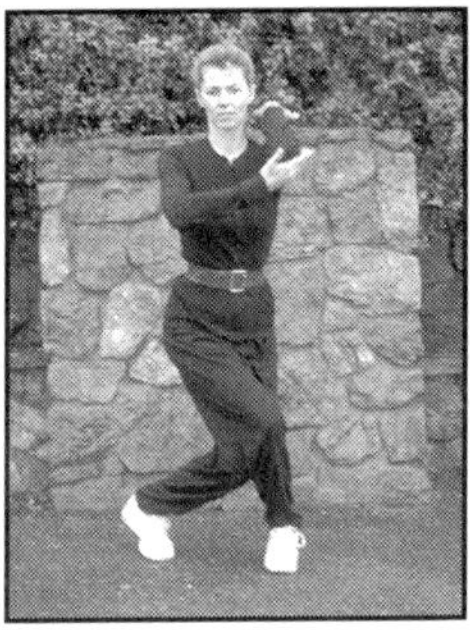

TwelveB

Lift the left knee and spread the hands to the sides while inhaling to the chest as shown in figure **Twelve A**.

Drop the left foot behind and to the right side of the right foot as you raise your left palm to the left shoulder and forcefully strike the left elbow with the right palm as you exhale to the Tan Tien as in figure **Twelve B**.

Repeat this stand-inhale drop-exhale sequence eight times.

Repeat the same sequence on the opposite side eight repetitions.

BODY SYSTEMS
Respiratory System, Circulatory System, Digestive System, Genito-Urinary System

PRIMARY CHANNELS
All

EXTRA-ORDINARY VESSELS
All By stimulation of their Master Points and Motion

YIN/YANG ORIENTATION
Balanced The stance moves from Yang to Yin and so do the arm positions.

EXTERNAL/INTERNAL
External The open palms collect Qi from nature and the upward movement collects Qi from the Earth through the standing leg.

ACUPUNCTURE POINTS
LI4, SI3, P6, P7, P8, LU7, LU9, TB4, TB5, HE7,by hand position TB10 by slapping under the elbow, GB21 by stimulating the top of shoulder, UB23,GV4 by turning of waist SP4, GB41, KI6, UB62 by foot position GV14, CV17 by expanding and contracting chest GB 21 is an important point in directing qi downwards in the body. In fact its downward function is so great that some systems use the point to collect Qi from Heaven. TB10 also descends rebellious Qi and has a special effect of the chest area. GV20 by mind regulation.

SPIRITUAL/ENERGETIC PROCESS
Standing on one leg while raising the other, spreading open palms to the sides and inhaling to the middle Tan Tien-chest-absorbs Earth Qi, environment Qi, and Heaven Qi to the Middle Tan Tien. Dropping and twisting one leg behind and to the outside of the other while exhaling to CV6 drives the Qi to the Lower Tan Tien. The patting of the elbow and shoulder encourage the Qi to descend. The twisting of the waist strongly activates the storage and transformative functions of the Kidney/Ming Men as well as stimulating the Belt Channel.

COMMENTARY
This exercise acts much like the Spinal Twist in Yoga, which is said to stimulate the Navel Chakra and digestive Fire (Ming Men).The overall effect of this exercise is that it gathers Qi from outside the body and concentrates the body's Qi in the Middle Tan Tien,then drives that concentration downwards to the Lower Tan Tien. Here again we have a packing activity. The left and right sides of the exercise open and harmonize the Left and Right Channels (Ming Men). This leaves the Lower Tan Tien packed with internal and external Qi and the transformative function of Ming Men activated—the perfect condition for the opening of the Central Channel.

Exercise Two

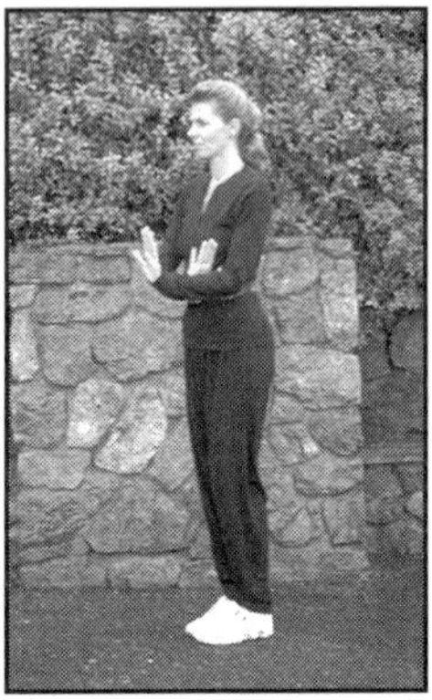

Twelve C

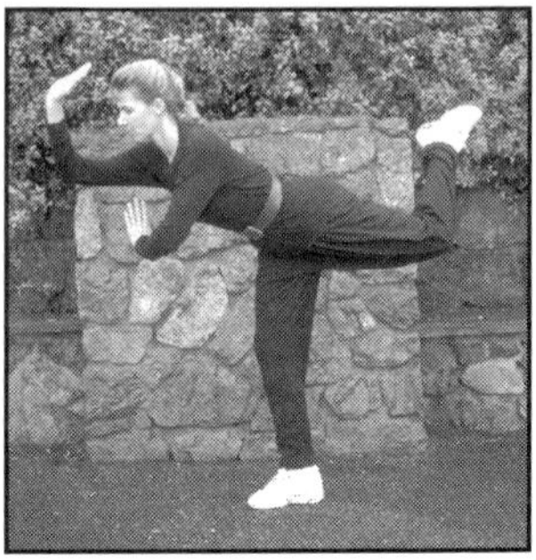

Twelve D

Stand with the left elbow touching the waist on the left side and the right palm facing the left elbow while inhaling to the Ming Men as in figure **Twelve C**.

Lean forward raising the right palm to the level of the head and pointing the fingertips of the left palm towards the right armpit. At the same time raise the left leg, bent at the knee with the toes pointing up, and exhale to the Tan Tien as in figure **Twelve D**.

Repeat this stand-inhale bend forward-exhale sequence eight times.

Do the same sequence eight times on the other side.

BODY SYSTEMS
All

PRIMARY CHANNELS
All

EXTRA-ORDINARY VESSELS
All

YIN/YANG ORIENTATION

Yang The stance is Yang, especially with one foot on the ground. The arms move from down to up and back down so have elements of both Yin and Yang.

EXTERNAL/INTERNAL

Internal Despite the open palms the main purpose to the exercise is to drive Qi up inside the body. There will be some interaction between the open top palm and the environment but mainly as a safety valve to protect against excess uprising Qi.

ACUPUNCTURE POINTS

LI4, SI3, P6, P7, P8,LU7, LU9, TB4, TB5, HE7, SP4, GB41, Ki6, UB62, GV4, UB23, CV6, HE1

SPIRITUAL/ENERGETIC PROCESS

Inhaling to Ming Men as the hands are placed in the starting position activates the Lower Tan Tien. Exhaling to CV6 as the leg is raised and the arms rise to the opposite side of the body pushes Qi upward. The arms crossing the body activate the Ming Men Channels, the bending forward activates Chong Mai. The level of the upper hand guides Qi to the top. The lower hand supports this Qi movement by activating HE1 on the opposite side through P9 and by channeling Qi to one side of the body. HE1 is one of the main points to open the flow of Qi to the arm.

COMMENTARY

Here again we have an upward mobilizing exercise following a lower gathering exercise with the transformative function of Ming Men as always playing a germane role.

Standing

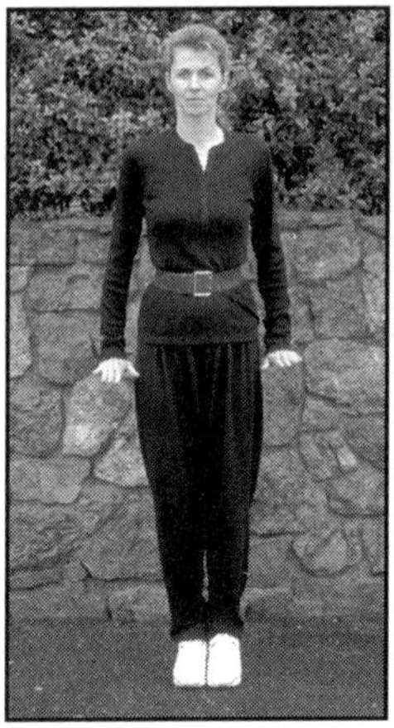

Twelve E

Stand with feet together hands at the sides with palms parallel to the ground as in figure **Twelve E**. Hold this position for eight breaths.

see Chapter Five Explanations

CHAPTER THIRTEEN *TIGER NEAR BODY*

The area between the thumb and the first finger is referred to as the Tigers Mouth. The name of his chapter points out the proximity of that area to the body in the exercises.

Exercise One

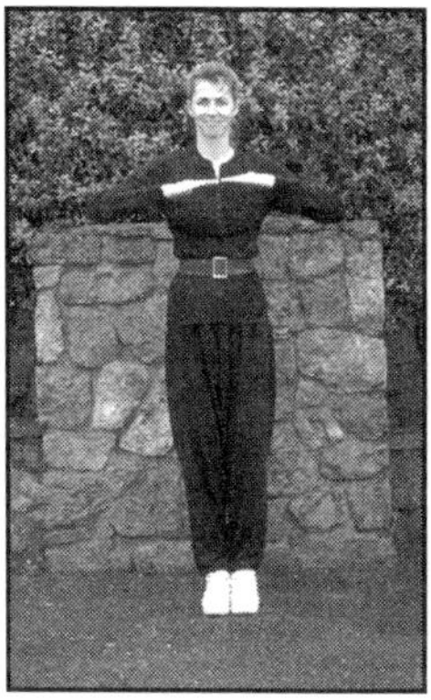

Thirteen A

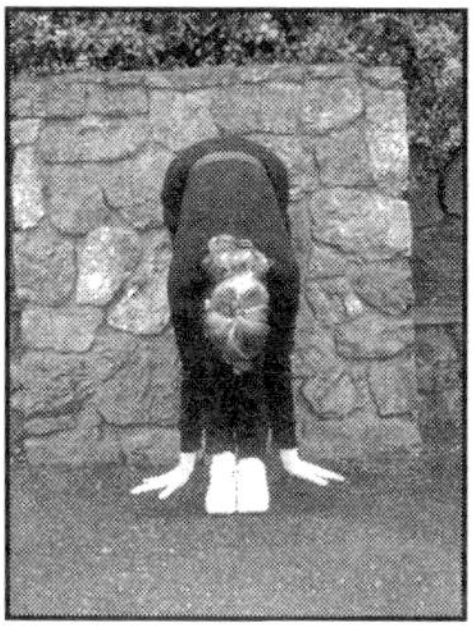

Thirteen B

Stand with feet together hands palm down and fingertips facing each other at chest level as in figure **Thirteen A** while inhaling to the chest.

Bend forward at the waist and extend the palms to the ground with a 180 degree twist while exhaling to the Tan Tien as in figure **Thirteen B**.

Turn palms upward and return to the position in figure **Thirteen A** while inhaling to the chest.

Repeat this bend-exhale raise-inhale sequence eight times.

BODY SYSTEMS
Respiratory System, Circulatory system, digestive System, Genito-Urinary System

PRIMARY CHANNELS—Lung Large Intestine, Heart Small Intestine, Pericardium, Triple Heater Urinary Bladder

EXTRA-ORDINARY VESSELS
Yin and Yang Wei by Master Points, Governing Vessel, Conception Vessel, Chong Mai Yin Chiao Mai by Master Points and body motion, Belt Channel by body motion'

YIN/YANG ORIENTATION
Yang Yang stance and balanced hand movements.

EXTERNAL/INTERNAL
External The Qi of Earth is absorbed and brought to the chest.

ACUPUNCTURE POINTS
SP4, KI6 by foot position GV4 UB23 by bending GV14 CV17 by expanding and contracting chest LI4. SI3, P6, P7, P8, TB4, TB5, LU7 ,LI9. HE7 by hand position KI1 by mind regulation

SPIRITUAL/ENERGETIC PROCESS
As the palms are brought up while inhaling, Qi from Earth is brought up to the chest. As the palms are lowered while exhaling to Cv6 part of the Qi from the Middle Tan Tien-chest-is collected in the Lower Tan Tien and part of the Qi returns to connect with Earth. The bending motion activates the storage and transformational functions of the Kidney/Ming Men.

COMMENTARY
This is a straight forward Earth Qi collecting exercise. Obviously it also increases circulation in the lower body and strengthens the lower back and Kidneys.

Exercise Two

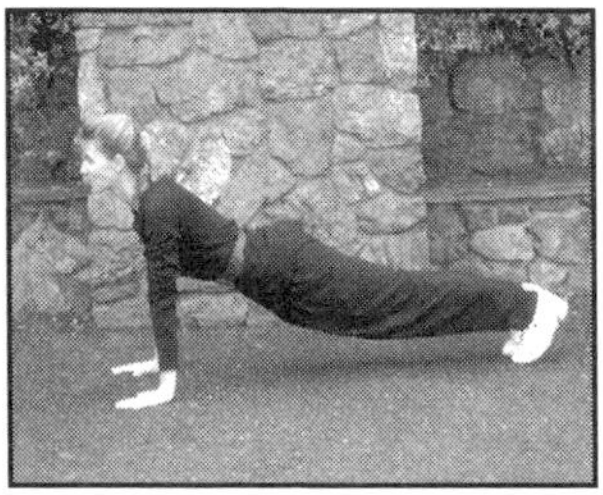

Thirteen C

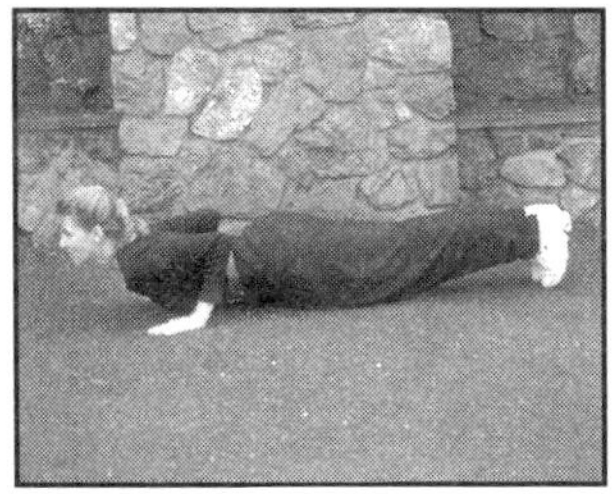

Thirteen D

Assume the traditional push-up position with head up as in figure **Thirteen C** while inhaling to the Ming Men.

Lower your body close to the ground without touching and exhale to the Tan Tien as in figure **Thirteen D**.

Repeat this exercise eight times.

BODY SYSTEMS
Respiratory System, Circulatory System

PRIMARY CHANNELS
Large intestine, Lung, Small Intestine, Heart, Triple Heater, Pericardium by movement, all the Leg channels by tension.

EXTRA-ORDINARY VESSELS—Yin and Yang Wei, Conception Vessel and Governing Vessel by hand position Chong Mai Belt Channel Yin and Yang Chiao Mai by foot position

YIN/YANG ORIENTATION
Yin Entire body is in Yin position and movement is close to the ground with Yin/Yang balance

EXTERNAL/INTERNAL

External Open palms on ground and Ki1 communicate with Earth Qi.

ACUPUNCTURE POINTS

CV17, GV14 by chest movement SP4, KI1, GB41, UB62, KI6 by foot position LI4, SI3, P6, P7, P8, TB4, TB5, LU7, LU8, HE7 by hand postion

SPIRITUAL/ENERGETIC PROCESS

As the body is pushed up while inhaling to the middle Tan Tien, Qi from Earth is absorbed to the chest from the arms and the legs. As the body is lowered while exhaling to CV6, the Qi from the Middle Tan Tien is stored in the Lower Tan Tien.

COMMENTARY

Another variation on the same theme except here all four major absorption points on the limbs are in direct contact with the ground. The head is held up to contain the flow of Qi to the Middle and Lower Tan Tiens.

Standing

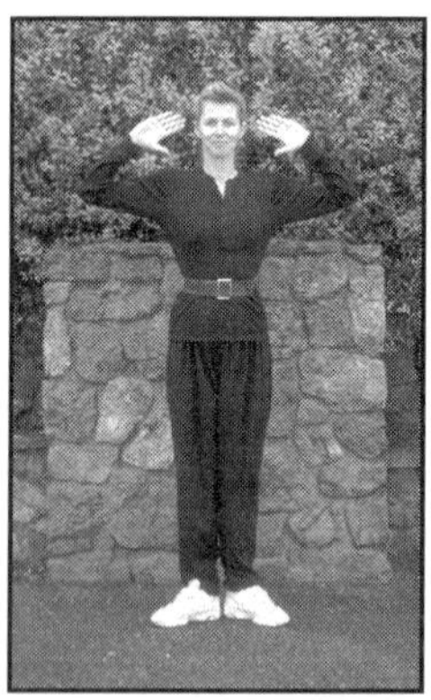

Thirteen E

Stand with the heels together with toes spread to form a straight toe-heel-heel-toe line. Bring the open palms up to point at the temple area of the head as in figure **Thirteen E**.

Hold this position for eight breaths.

BODY SYSTEMS
Circulatory System, Digestive System, Respiratory System

PRIMARY CHANNELS
All

EXTRA-ORDINARY VESSELS
Governing Vessel, Conception Vessel, Yin and yang Wei Mai by hand position, Chong Mai and Yin Chiao Mai by foot position'

YIN/YANG ORIENTATION
Yang Stance and arms are in a Yang mode.

EXTERNAL/INTERNAL
Internal Palms are open but Qi is directed to head.

ACUPUNCTURE POINTS
SP4, KI6 by foot position LI4, SI3, P6, P7, P8, LU7, LU9, TB4, TB5, HE7 by hand position P9 by mind regulation

SPIRITUAL/ENERGETIC PROCESS
The body position leads the Qi stored in the Lower Tan Tien up to the head with special emphasis focused because the Qi emitted from the two P9 points directs the Qi to the Upper Tan Tien (Brow Chakra).

COMMENTARY
Another gather the Qi in the Lower Tan Tien and bring it up to the head chapter.

CHAPTER FOURTEEN *CONFINE CIRCULAR FORCE*

The first two exercises of this chapter are more difficult versions of earlier exercises. The earlier exercises utilized more confined up and down movements to move the Qi. In Chapter Fourteen, the movements of these two exercises are much bigger and more stretched out, parts of which resemble a circle. The expertise required in these techniques is to concentrate that bigger movement into the internal focus of the exercise.

Exercise One

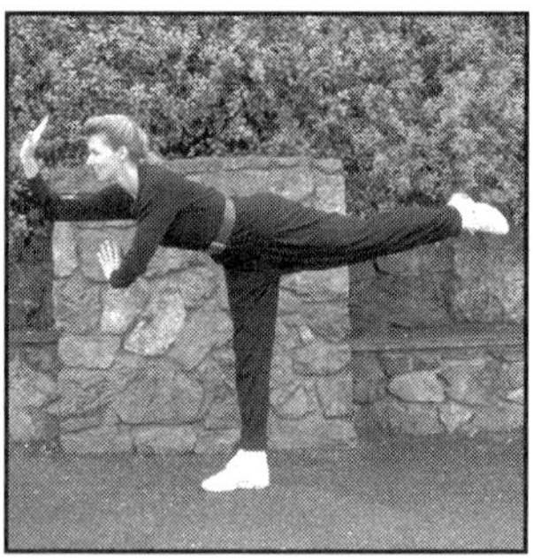

Fourteen A

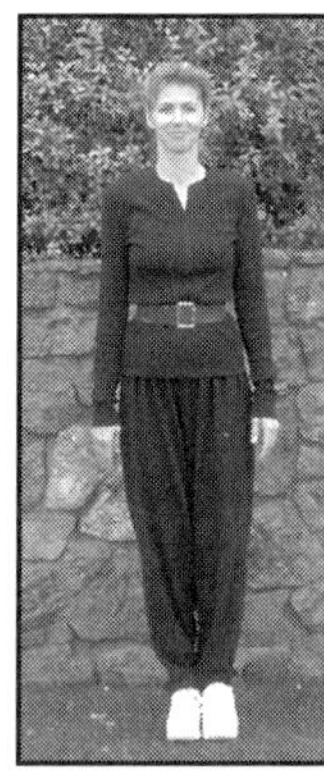

Fourteen B

From a standing position stretch the left leg straight back parallel to the ground, lean forward, raise the right palm slightly higher than the head, and push the left palm, fingers up, under the right armpit while exhaling to the Tan Tien as in figure **Fourteen A**.

Return to the standing position inhaling to the Ming Men as in figure **Forteeen B**.

Stretch the right leg straight back parallel to the ground, lean forward, raise the left palm slightly higher than the head, and push the right palm, fingers up, under the right armpit while exhaling to the Tan Tien.

Return to the standing position inhaling to the Ming Men.

Perform this right-left sequence eight times.

BODY SYSTEMS
All

PRIMARY CHANNELS
All

EXTRA-ORDINARY VESSELS
All

YIN/YANG ORIENTATION
Yang   The stance is Yang, especially with one foot on the ground. The arms move from down to up and back down so have elements of both Yin and Yang.

EXTERNAL/INTERNAL
Internal   Despite the open palms the main purpose to the exercise is to drive Qi up inside the body. There will be some interaction between the open top palm and the environment but mainly as a safety valve to protect against excess uprising Qi.

ACUPUNCTURE POINTS
LI4, SI3, P6, P7, P8,LU7, LU9, TB4, TB5, HE7, SP4, GB41, Ki6, UB62, GV4, UB23, CV6, HE1

SPIRITUAL/ENERGETIC PROCESS
Inhaling to Ming Men in the starting position activates the Lower Tan Tien. Exhaling to CV6 as the leg is raised and the arms rise to the opposite side of the body pushes Qi upward. The arms crossing the body activate the Ming Men Channels, the bending forward activates Chong Mai. The level of the upper hand guides Qi to the top. The lower hand supports this Qi movement by activating HE1 on the opposite side through P9 and by channeling Qi to one side of the body. HE1 is one of the main points to open the flow of Qi to the arm.

COMMENTARY
Here again we have an upward mobilizing exercise.

see Chapter Twelve, Exercise Two

Exercise Two

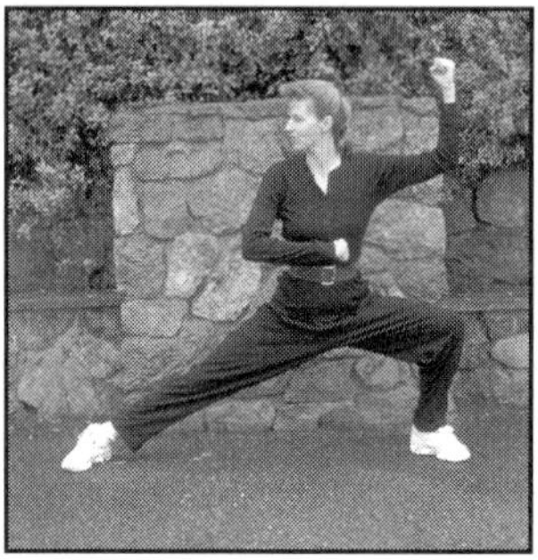

Fourteen C

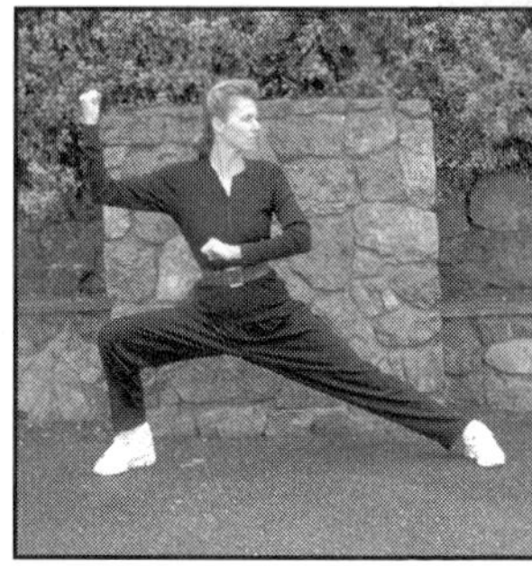

Fourteen D

Stretch the right leg far to the right side, bend the left knee, raise the left hand slightly higher than the head, and cross the right fist to the left side of the body while inhaling to the chest as in figure **Fourteen C**.

Then switch the entire posture to the opposite side as in figure **Fourteen D**. Exhale to the Tan Tien as the hands meet in the center and inhale to the chest as the left hand rises above the left hand.

Perform this right-left sequence eight times and return to standing.

BODY SYSTEMS
Respiratory System, Circulatory System, Digestive System, Genito-Urinary System

PRIMARY CHANNELS
All

EXTRA-ORDINARY VESSELS
Yin and Yang Chiao Mai, Chong Mai and Belt Channel by foot positions. The up and down motion of the hands stimulates Conception Vessel as it takes place in line with and close to the Channel. Up and down motion always tends to stimulate the Conception and Governing Vessels and Chong Mai.

YIN/YANG ORIENTATION

Yin   The stance is Yin (modulate by the toe up movement) and the arm movements are not large nor extended above the head. Even though the focus of this exercise is to move Qi up and down, the overall construction of the form is Yin. Here we have a case of exercising the Yang in Yin.

EXTERNAL/INTERNAL

Internal   The hands remaining "closed" keep the focus of this exercise internal, although there is some interaction with the Earth.

ACUPUNCTURE POINTS

UB62, KIL, SP4, GB41 by foot position CV6 and GV4 by breath GV4 and UB23 by side to side waist and arm raising motion CV17 by fists crossing close and GV14 BY alternate arm raising.

SPIRITUAL/ENERGETIC PROCESS

As we inhale and raise the fist, the Qi is moved subtly but powerfully up the Right or Left Side Channel—Ming Men— to the head, The lower fist keeps the Qi channeled to one side of the body or the other. The fist moving to center as the body starts to descend concentrates the Qi in the Upper Tan Tien-Brow Chakra- before descending down the Conception Vessel .

COMMENTARY

Both exercises in this chapter are high level and quite subtle. Dealing with the Yin in Yang and the Yang in Yin is a delicate and a very profound experience.

Exercise Three

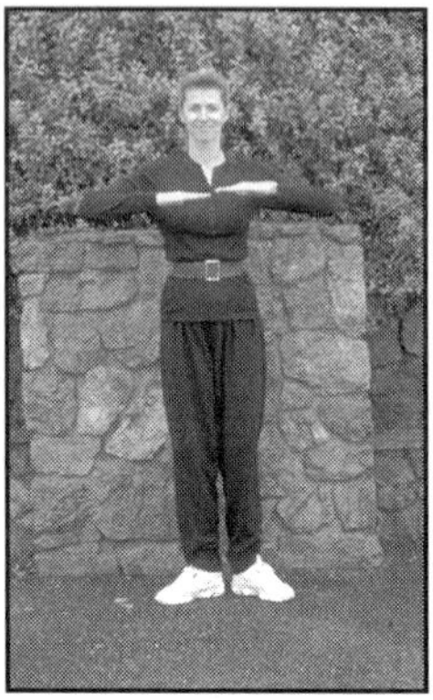

Fourteen E

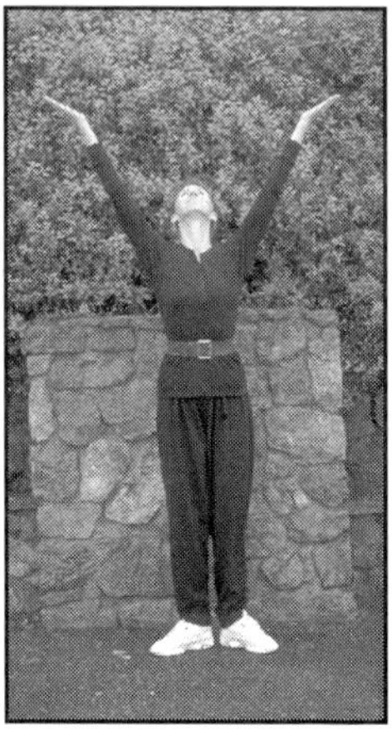

Fourteen F

Stand with heels together toes spread apart (v shaped) and open palms at chest level as in figure **Fourteen E**.

Raise the palms overhead with fingertips pointing to the sides as in figure **Fourteen F**, while inhaling to the chest.

Return the palms to the chest as in figure **Fourteen E** exhaling to the Tan Tien.

Perform this raising-inhale lower-exhale sequence eight times.

BODY SYSTEMS
Respiratory, Circulatory, Digestive

PRIMARY CHANNELS
ALL

EXTRA-ORDINARY VESSELS
ALL

YIN/YANG ORIENTATION
Yang The stance is Yang and the arm position is Yang

EXTERNAL/INTERNAL
External The open palms and feet allow free communication with nature.

ACUPUNCTURE POINTS
LI4, SI3,P6, P7, P8, LU7, LU9, TB4, TB5, HE7 by hand position CV17, GV14 by expansion and contraction of chest, KI6, UB62 by foot position Yin Tang, GV20 by mind regulation CV6, GV4 and CV17 by breath

SPIRITUAL/ENERGETIC PROCESS
Raising the hands, looking partially up, and feeling up to the sky while inhaling to the Middle Tan Tien connects man with Heaven. Bringing the hands and head down and feeling into the Lower Tan Tien while exhaling to CV6 brings the Qi of Heaven into man to be stored in the Lower Tan Tien

COMMENTARY
The previous two exercises focused Qi in the Upper Tan Tien—"nourishing the Spirit". This exercise joins the Spirit with Heaven-God-Tao-etc.

Standing

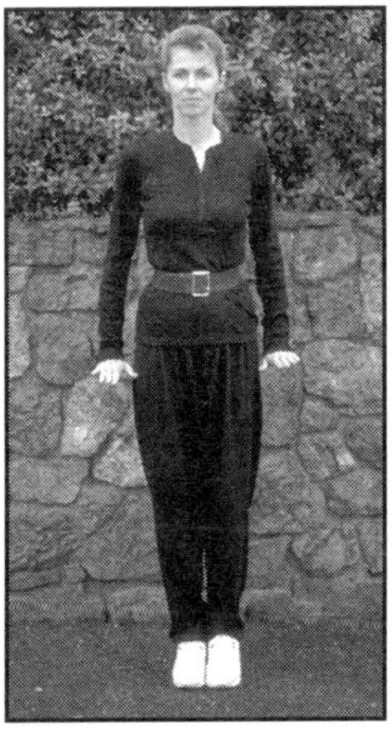

Fourteen G

Stand with feet together, hands at the sides with palms parallel to the ground as in figure **Fourteen G**. Hold this position for eight breaths.

see Chapter Five Explanations

CHAPTER FIFTEEN *FATHER AND SON SALUTE*

The title of this chapter originally referred to the first exercise where one hand is a fist (father-Yang) and the other hand is open yet pointing up and in direct connection with the fist (son-less Yang). With the addition of the new exercise the name still fits as we have one exercise with two fists (father-Yang) and one exercise with one fist and one open hand (son-less Yang).

Exercise One

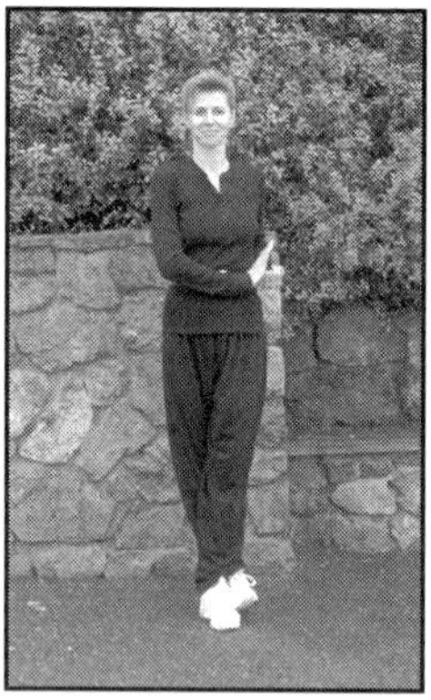

Fifteen A

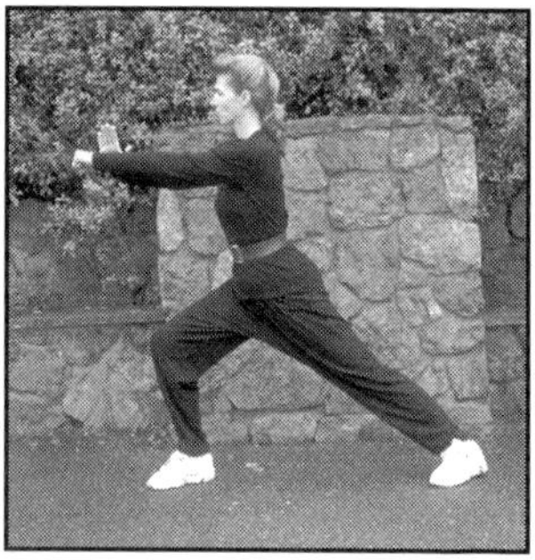

Fifteen B

Move the right foot behind and to the left side of the left foot and rest it on its heel. Place the left fist with the palm facing upward at the left side at waist level and place the right forearm across the abdomen with the palm facing the left fist as in figure **Fifteen A**.

Step the right foot to the right side with knee bent while extending the left leg and pushing the left fist out at shoulder level while inhaling to the Ming Men. The right palm will follow the left fist to end resting on the left wrist as in figure **Fifteen B**.

Return to the position pictured in **Fifteen A** while exhaling to the Tan Tien.

Perform this step in and out sequence eight times.

Now perform this sequence eight times on the other side.

BODY SYSTEMS
Respiratory System, Circulatory System, Digestive System Genito-urinary System

PRIMARY CHANNELS
All

EXTRA-ORDINARY VESSELS
All

YIN/YANG ORIENTATION
Balance The stance is Yin and the hands are neutral but the Yin stance is balanced by Yang movement.

EXTERNAL/INTERNAL
Internal The open palm is directed back towards the arm of the practitioner.

ACUPUNCTURE POINTS
LI4, SI3, P6, P7, P8, LU7, LU9, TB4, TB5, HE7 by hand position, GB26 by hands at waist postion UB23 AND GV4 by waist turn GV4, CV6, CV17 by breath GV14, CV17 by chest expansion and contraction KI6, UB62, GB41, SP4 by foot position

SPIRITUAL/ENERGETIC PROCESS
Stepping out, thrusting one fist out with the opposite palm facing the wrist area while inhaling to the Middle Tan Tien brings Qi up the Ming Men (left or Right Side Channels) Channel to the level of the shoulder. The closed fist allows the Qi to fill thc arm and not dissipate outside. The open palm directs Qi from that side of the body to the fist side. P8 in the palm activates LU7 on the wrist to open the Conception Vessel which facilitates the return of Qi to the Lower Tan Tien. Returning to the starting position and exhaling to CV6 returns the Qi to the Lower Tan Tien. The Governing Vessel is also stimulated in the begining position by P8 on the palm facing SI3

COMMENTARY
This exercise pumps the Ming Men Channels full of transformed Qi from the Lower Tan Tien and opens the Conception Vessel to help cool and balance the body.

Exercise Two

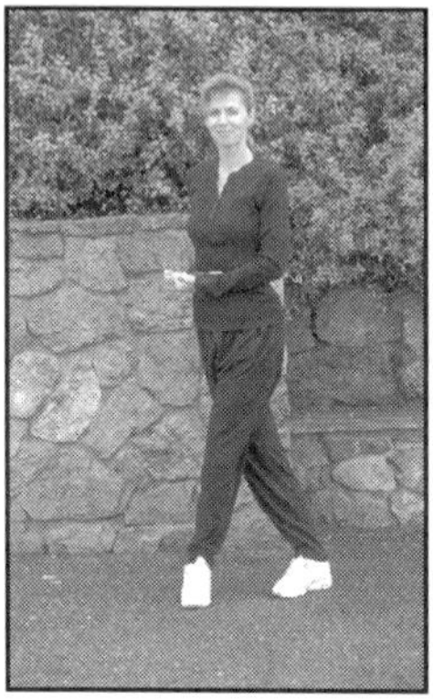

Fifteen C

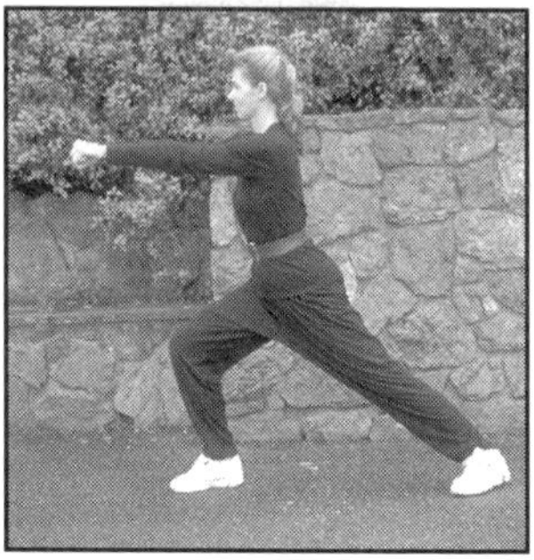

Fifteen D

Place the right foot behind and far to the left side of the left foot resting fully on the sole. Hold both fists, palm up, at the right side of the body waist high as in figure **Fifteen C** while inhaling to the Ming Men.

Step to the right with the right foot straightening the left leg and bending the right knee as you extend both fists out to shoulder height while exhaling to the Tan Tien as in figure **Fifteen D**.

Return to the position pictured in **Fifteen C**.

Repeat this step out-exhale step in-inhale sequence eight times.

Change positions and repeat the same exercise eight times on the other side.

BODY SYSTEMS
All

PRIMARY CHANNELS
All

EXTRA-ORDINARY VESSELS
All

YIN/YANG ORIENTATION

Yang The stances and hands are both Yin and Yang but there is lots of movement.

EXTERNAL/INTERNAL

Internal/External Both hands are in fists. There is an Earth connection as both feet are on the ground, primarily as a method of using Earth Qi to balance the large amount of Qi in the arms and upper body. Qi from both Heaven and Earth is also drawn in and excess Qi is expelled through GV20 and KiL.

ACUPUNCTURE POINTS

same as above except for the P8-Lu7 connection

SPIRITUAL/ENERGETIC PROCESS

Inhaling to the Ming Men while assuming the beginning position draws Qi from earth and heaven to be absorbed and concentrate in the Lower Tan Tien, Exhaling to CV6 while stepping out and thrusting fists forward at shoulder level moves this mixed and transformed Qi up both Ming Men channels and out to the fists. GV20 is opened as a safety valve by Mind Regulation.

COMMENTARY

In this powerful exercise Fire and Water Qi from the Middle Tan Tien and Lower Tan Tien supplemented by Yin and Yang Qi from Earth and Heaven are mixed, transformed, and used to pump the Ming Men Channels.

Standing

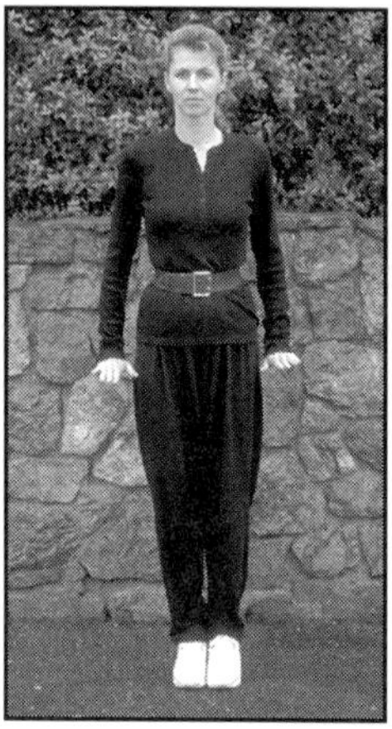

Fifteen E

Stand with feet together hands at the sides with palms parallel to the ground as in figure **Fifteen E.**

see Chapter Five Explanations

CHAPTER SIXTEEN *FLUTTERING CARP*

Fluttering Carp refers to the movement of the first exercise in the chapter. The exercise actually has the practitioner emersed in Yin Qi from Earth much as a Fluttering Carp is emersed in water.

Exercise One

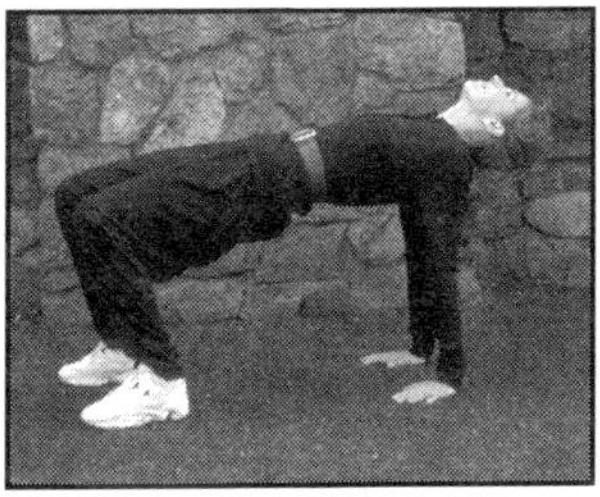

Sixteen A

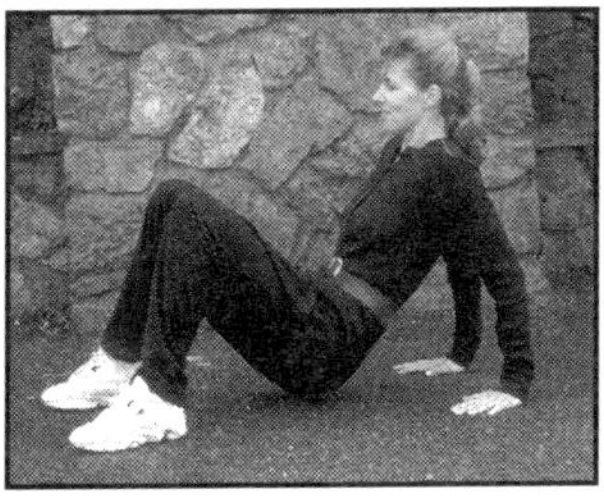

Sixteen B

Assume the "crab" position inhaling to the Ming Men as in figure **Sixteen A**.

Lower the hips to the ground exhaling to the Tan Tien as in figure **Sixteen B**.

Perform this up-inhale down-exhale sequence eight times.

BODY SYSTEMS
Circulatory , Digestive, Respiratory, Genito-Urinary

PRIMARY CHANNELS
All

EXTRA-ORDINARY VESSELS
All

YIN/YANG ORIENTATION
Yin Stance is Yin and both hands and feet are connected to the ground.

EXTERNAL/INTERNAL

External Both hands and feet draw Yin Qi from the Earth.

ACUPUNCTURE POINTS

LI4, SI3, P6, P7, P8, LU7, LU9, TB4, TB5, HE7 by hand position GV4 and CV6 by breath and movement UB23 by movement P8 and KiL by mind regulation GV14 and CV17 by expansion and contraction of chest.

SPIRITUAL/ENERGETIC PROCESS

Inhaling to Ming Men and raising the body with mind regulation gathers Yin Qi from Earth through both the hands and feet. Lowering the body while exhaling to CV6 stores the Yin Qi in the Lower Tan Tien. The upward and downward motions of the body activate the storage and transformational functions of the Kidney/Ming Men. With weight on the hands and feet, the upward and downward motions combined with the expansion and contraction of the abdomen balance Blood and Qi in the whole body.

COMMENTARY

Like a Carp in water, the practitioner is emersed in Yin Qi in this exercise.

Exercise Two

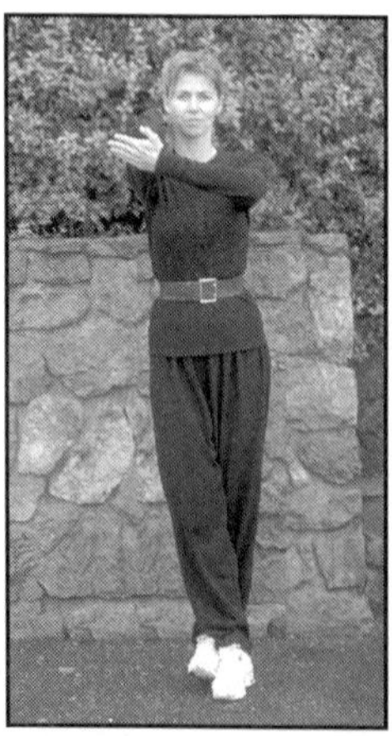

Sixteen C

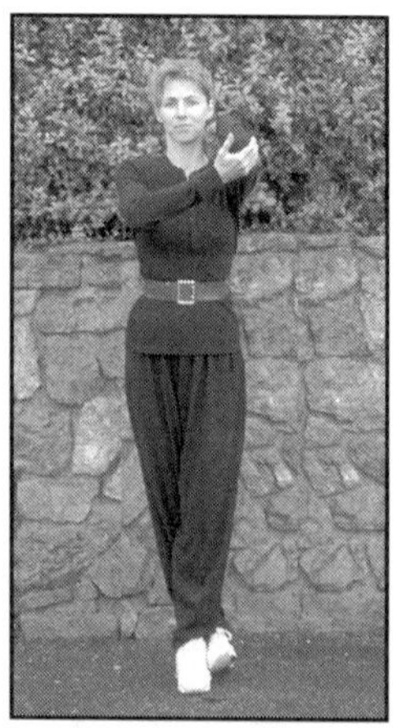

Sixteen D

Move the left foot behind and to the right side of the right foot, touching the ground with the left heel and hooking the left toes on top of the right foot. At the same time, raise the right fist to the right shoulder and slap under the right elbow with the left palm forcefully as you inhale to the Ming Men as in figure **Sixteen C**.

Return to standing as you exhale to the Tan Tien.

Move the right foot behind and to the left side of the left foot, touching the ground with the right heel and hooking the right toes on top of the left foot. At the same time raise the left fist to the left shoulder and slap under the left elbow with the right palm forcefully as you inhale to the Ming Men as in figure **Sixteen D**.

Return to standing as you exhale to the Tan Tien.

Perform this right-left sequence eight times.

BODY SYSTEMS
Circulatory, Respiratory, Digestive, Genito-Urinary

PRIMARY CHANNELS
All

EXTRA-ORDINARY VESSELS
All

YIN/YANG ORIENTATION
Yang   The stance is Yang and the arm movement is Yang.

EXTERNAL/INTERNAL
Internal   The hands are closed and only one foot is on the ground.

ACUPUNCTURE POINTS
GB41, KI6, SP4, UB62 by foot positions TB10 and P8 by slapping CV6, GV4 by breath LI4, SI3, P6, P7, P8, TB4, GB21, TB5, LU7, LU9, HE7 by hand position CV17 and GV14 by expansion and contraction of chest UB23 and GV4 by side to side motion

SPIRITUAL/ENERGETIC PROCESS
Inhaling to the Middle Tan Tien while crossing the leg and raising fist to shoulder brings Qi up the Ming Men channel (left or right side channels). Slapping TB10 activates its descending and spirit calming functions thus

accenting one sided Qi flow and Qi packing in the channel. GB21 is stimulated by close proximity of the fist to supplement action of TB10. Exhaling to the Lower Tan Ten while returning to the starting position returns Qi to the Lower Tan Tien.

Standing

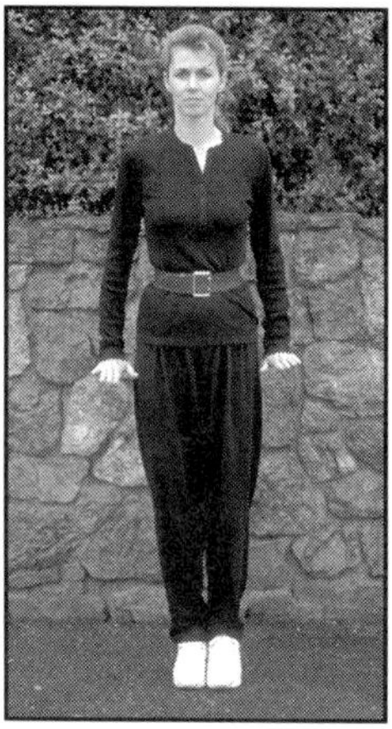

Sixteen E

Stand with feet together hands at the sides with palms facing and parallel to the ground as in figure **Sixteen E.**

Hold this position for eight breaths.

see Chapter Five Explanations

CHAPTER SEVENTEEN *JUNG LI PRESENTS CAPE*

The movement in the first exercise is somewhat like putting on a cape. When an advanced practitioner performs this exercise the Qi flow up the back can be so full that it feels like a cape is covering the back.

Exercise One

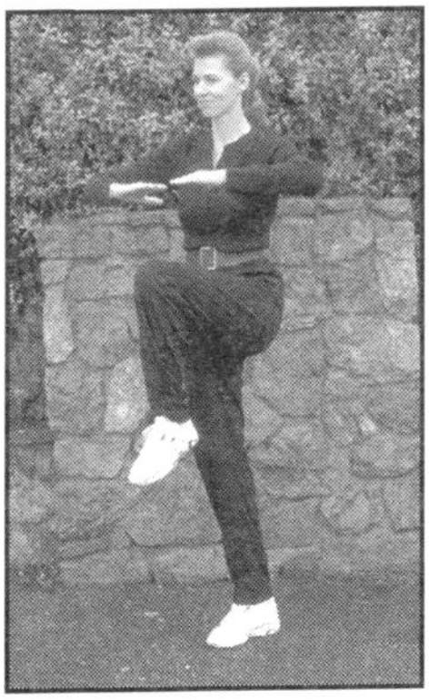

Seventeen A

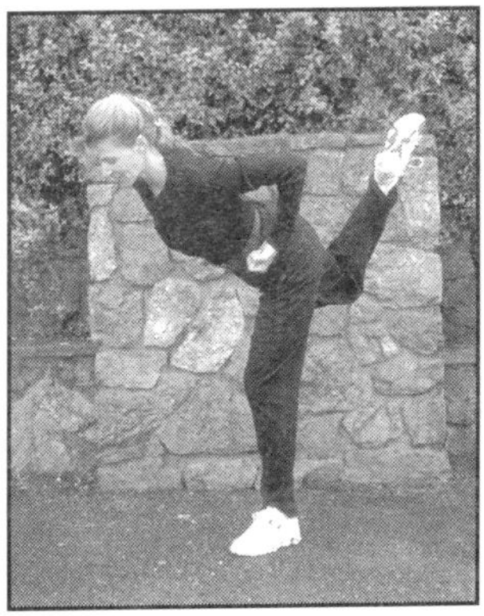

Seventeen B

Lift the left knee high and bring both palms up behind the midline of the body, past the ears, and down to the level of the heart as in figure **Seventeen A** while inhaling to the Ming Men.

Lower the left foot to the ground and raise the right leg with the knee bent as you bend slightly forward and place your fists at your waist while exhaling to the Tan Tien as in figure **Seventeen B**.

Repeat this sequence eight times.

Change positions and repeat this exercise eight times on the other side.

BODY SYSTEMS
Respiratory, Circulatory, Digestive, Genito-Urinary

PRIMARY CHANNELS
All

EXTRA-ORDINARY VESSELS
All

YIN/YANG ORIENTATION
Yang The stances are all more Yang due to single leg and slight bending and the hand movements are balanced between upward and downward.

EXTERNAL/INTERNAL
External Qi from the Earth is brought up through the body by mind regulation and movement. Heaven Qi is also absorb through GV20

ACUPUNCTURE POINTS
LI4, SI3, P6, P7, P8, LU7, LU9, TB4, TB5, HE7 by hand position UB62, KI6, SP4, GB41 by foot position GV14, CV17 by chest expansion and contraction UB23, GV4 by waist bending GV4,CV6 by breath GB26 by fists at waist GV20 by Mind Regulation

SPIRITUAL/ENERGETIC PROCESS
Inhaling to CV17 while raising one leg and moving the arms up and to the front brings Qi from the Earth through the leg, up the back, over the head and down to the Middle Tan Tien and Heaven Qi via GV20 is also added by Mind Regulation. Exhaling to the Lower Tan Tien while lowering the hands in fists to the waist and changing legs moves the Qi to the Lower Tan Tien and back to the ground. This completes the famous Big Heavenly Circle of circulating Qi in all the Extra-Ordinary Vessels.

COMMENTARY
This exercise not only completes the Big Heavenly Circle (sometimes call Big Earth or the Macro-Cosmic Orbit) but alternates the lower routes leg to leg which pumps the Ming Men Channels-Ida and Pingala-Left and Right Channels and harmonizes them. This harmony is necessary for the Chong Mai-Central Channel-Sushumi- to open. When an adept performs the exercise his back will truly be cloaked in transformed Qi.

Exercise Two

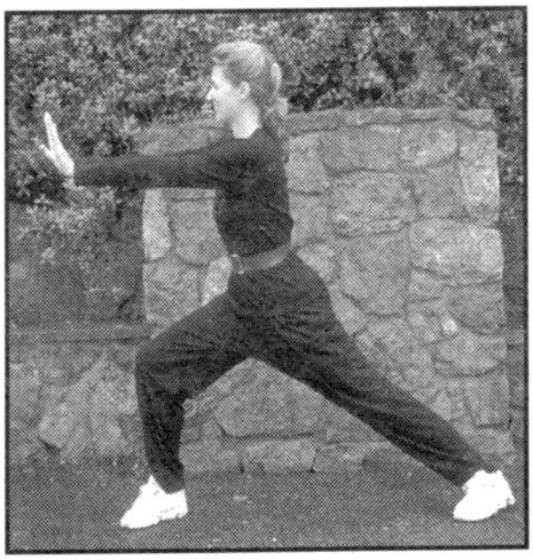

Seventeen C

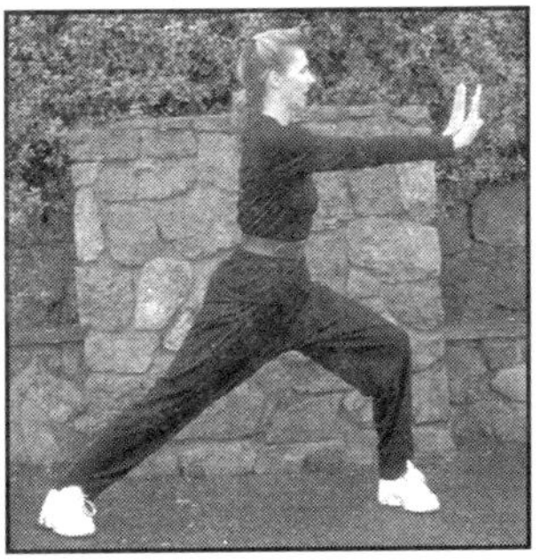

Seventeen D .

Move the right leg to the right side with bent knee while extending the left leg. At the same time push both palms evenly to the right side exhaling to the Tan Tien as in figure **Seventeen C**.

Turn to face forward with palms facing your heart inhaling to the Ming Men.

Now turn to the left and put both palms evenly out to the left while exhaling to the Tan Tien as in figure **Seventeen D**.

Push right and left eight times (to each side).

BODY SYSTEMS
Respiratory , Circulatory, Digestive, Genito-Urinary

PRIMARY CHANNELS
All

EXTRA-ORDINARY VESSELS
All

YIN/YANG ORIENTATION
Balanced   The stance is Yin but moving which adds a Yang quality and the arms are balanced.

EXTERNAL/INTERNAL

External The open palms communicate with nature

ACUPUNCTURE POINTS

see above except for fists at waist and bending

SPIRITUAL/ENERGETIC PROCESS

Exhaling to the Lower Tan Tien while turning and pushing the palms out gathers Qi in the lower Tan Tien and pushes it to the extremities, both feet and hands. The open palms allow any excess to be dispersed to the exterior. Inhaling to Ming Men while returning the palms to the front of the chest gathers Qi to the Lower Tan Tien and balances the Heart.

COMMENTARY

The first exercise in this chapter is very powerfully invigorating. The second exercise allows the body to balance itself and harmonize with the environment.

Standing

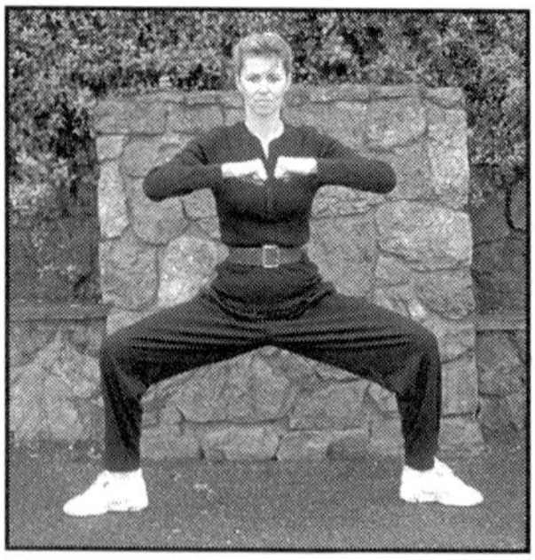

Seventeen E

Spread the legs and bend both knees with the toes pointed half way to the sides. Hold both fists at heart level with the palms facing down as in figure **Seventeen E**.

Hold this position eight breaths.

BODY SYSTEMS
Respiratory, Circulatory

Primary Channels
All

EXTRA-ORDINARY VESSELS
All

YIN/YANG ORIENTATION
Yin Yin stance and neutral arms

EXTERNAL/INTERNAL
Internal No active interaction with nature

ACUPUNCTURE POINTS
GV14 is opened by position of back, CV17 is stimulated by proximity to LI4 and HE1 is opened by arm position. The only unusual Acupoint combination here is the relationship of LI4 to CV17. LI4 can adjust the Qi transformation functions of the whole body thus increasing its natural healing power. It also has a special influence on the brain. Being on the Large Intestine Channel LI4, is especially useful for increasing movement below the navel, in the Lower Sea of Qi. CV17, called the Upper Sea of Qi, is the meeting point of all the Qi of the body.

SPIRITUAL/ENERGETIC PROCESS
The legs are bent and turned out halfway, allowing free circulation in the lower extremities. The arms are circled in front which usually increases circulation in the Middle Tan Tien but the hands are in fists allowing, but not inducing circulation. The position allows the Qi to stabilize itself at a deep level in the entire body

COMMENTARY
In this chapter we have the first exercise to strongly mobilize Qi , the second to allow the body to find balance in movement and the standing to allow the body to find balance in stillness.

CHAPTER EIGHTEEN
HANG BOTTLE WITH GOLDEN HOOK

The body is often regarded as a bottle-to fill with transformed Qi—Golden Elixir. The process for producing the elixir is to put Qi from the Middle Tan Tien under Qi from the Lower Tan Tien—mix the two Qi's and utilize the transformative function of Ming Men to "fire" the mixture to form the "Elixir of Immortality". The hands in this exercise ,being representatives of the Middle Tan Tien, hook the feet, which are representatives of the Lower Tan Tien. The Golden Elixir can then be produced through energetic transformation.

Exercise One

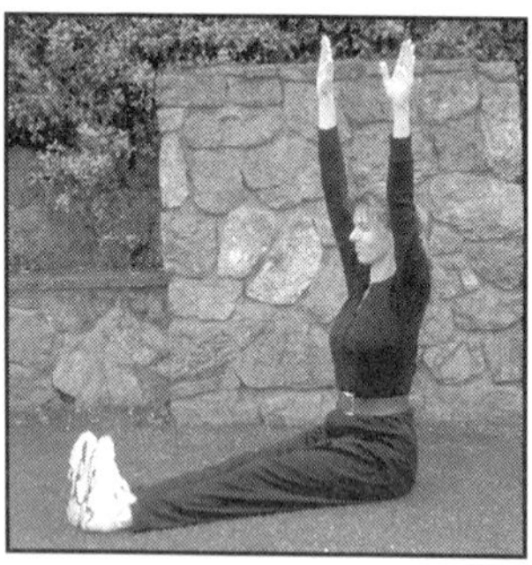

Eighteen A

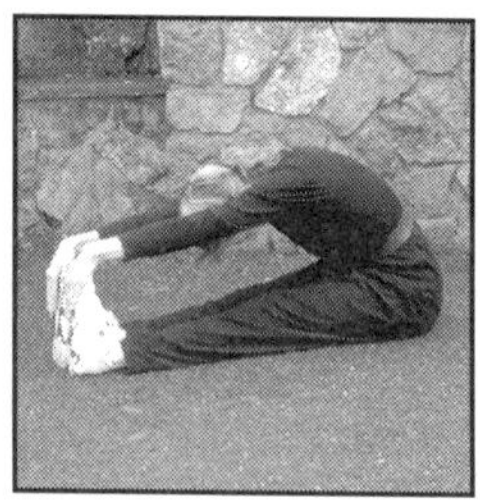

Eighteen B

Sit on the floor with the legs outstretched and hands held above the head as in figure **Eighteen A** while inhaling to the Middle Tan Tien.

Bend at the waist and extend your palms over the top of the foot while exhaling to the Tan Tien as in figure **Eighteen B**.

Repeat this sit up-inhale bend over-exhale eight times.

BODY SYSTEMS
Respiratory, Circulatory, Digestive, Genito-Urinary

PRIMARY CHANNELS
All are stretched.

EXTRA-ORDINARY VESSELS
Chong Mai, Conception Vessel, Governing Vessel and Belt Vessel by movement. All by Master Points

YIN/YANG ORIENTATION
Balance Yin stance by legs on the ground and Yang Hands by upraised position. Movement is balanced.

EXTERNAL/INTERNAL
Internal Major external communication points are joined to each other.

ACUPUNCTURE POINTS
KI6, P8 by proximity LI4, SI3, P6, P7, P8, LU7, LU9, TB4, TB5, HE7 by hand position GV4, UB23 by waist bending, SP4, GB41, UB62,KI6 by foot position GV4 and CV6 by breath

SPIRITUAL/ENERGETIC PROCESS
Inhaling to Middle Tan Tien while raising arms up brings Qi from Lower Tan Tien to Middle Tan Tien . Exhaling to Lower Tan Tien while bringing arms down to connect with feet brings Qi from Middle Tan Tien down to the Lower Tan Tien. This mixes the two Qis as does the direct connection of P8 in the Palms with Ki1 on the soles. The exercise mixes and balances Fire and Water, The bending and raising of the waist stimulates the storage and transformative functions of the Kidney/Ming Men and induces the mixed "Elixir" to ascend the Chong Mai within the spine.

COMMENTARY
The mixing and transformation of fire and water in man refines the individual energies. The next step is to merge with the One.

Standing

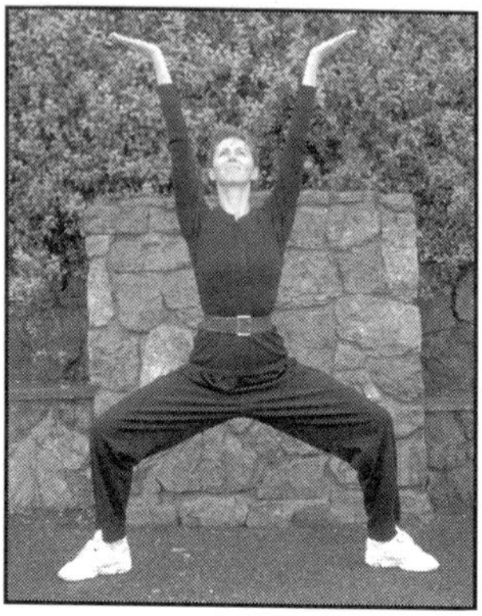

Eighteen C

Spread the legs and toes apart while bending the knees. Hold both hands above the shoulders and point the fingers of the open palms to the sides as in figure **Eighteen C**. Look slightly up.

Hold this position eight breaths.

This concludes the Eighteen Buddha Hands QiGong.

BODY SYSTEMS
All

PRIMARY CHANNELS
All

EXTRA-ORDINARY VESSELS
All

YIN/YANG ORIENTATION
Balanced Yin legs and Yang arms

EXTERNAL/INTERNAL
One

ACUPUNCTURE POINTS

SI3, P8, P7, P6, LU7, LU9, TB4, TB5, HE7, CV17, GV14, SP4, KI6

SP4 and Ki6 Master points of Chong Mai and Yin Chiao Mai are opened by the spreading of the feet to the sides. P8, the major point of communication between man and nature on the upper extremities, is opened by the spreading palms and hand position as are the points SI3, P6, P7, LU7, LU9, TB4, TB5, HE7, CV17, and GV14. SI3 is the Master Point of the Governing Vessel, P6 is the Master Point of Yin Wei Mai, LU7 is the Master Point of the Conception Vessel, TB5 is the Master Point of Yang Wei Mai, P7 and HE7 are points that regulate the Heart and bring Peace and Harmony to the Spirit. LU9 is the reunion point of the energy that moves the blood in the vessels of the entire body, GV14 is the meeting point of all the Yang Channels in the body and a major point to strengthen defensive energy, and CV17 is the meeting point of the Qi of the body.

SPIRITUAL/ENERGETIC PROCESS

The feet are in a stance conducive to unrestricted Qi flow in either direction, as are the arms. This stance offers the possibility of direct communication between Heaven and Earth through Man. It all depends on the MIND.

COMMENTARY

If the mind is regulated beyond regulation—empty- the possibilities are

UNLIMITED !

APPENDIX A ACUPUNCTURE POINTS

A body inch is the width of the interphalangeal joint of the thumb.

Lung (LU) 7—Broken Sequence
Location—1.5 body inches above the wrist crease in a depression at the origin of the styloid process
Functions—OPENS AND REGULATES the Conception Vessel, releases exterior conditions and expels wind, regulates the Lungs, activates the Lung Channel and alleviates pain.

LU 9—Great Abyss
Location—In a depression at the radial end of the wrist crease.
Functions—Regulates and tonifies the Lungs, eliminates wind and transforms phlegm, MEETING POINT OF THE BLOOD VESSELS.

Large Intestine (LI) 4—Joining Valley
Location—On the back of the hand between the 1st and 2nd metacarpal bones close to the radial border of the midpoint of the second metacarpal bone.
Functions—Relieves exterior conditions and expels wind, TONIFIES AND REGULATES DEFENSIVE QI, balances sweating, clears channels, regulates eyes, ears, nose, mouth, alleviates pain, restores Yang, regulates Lung and Large Intestine, softens hard masses, relaxes sinews, promotes labor.

Spleen (SP) 4—Grandfather Grandson
Location—At the junction of the red and white skin in a depression one body inch behind the joint of the big toe.
Functions—REGULATES CHONG MAI, Regulates Spleen and Stomach, Tonifies Source Qi, clears heat, benefits Heart and chest, transforms phlegm, calms the Spirit, clears the brain, invigorates blood.

SP 10—Sea of Blood
Location—Two Body Units superior to the medial superior border of the Patella.
Functions—INVIGORATES, REGULATES, AND TONIFIES BLOOD; clears stasis, cools blood, harmonizes menstruation, regulates the Spleen.

Heart (HE) 1— Summits Spring

Location—In a depression at the center of the armpit medial to the axially artery
Functions—Regulates the Heart, expands and relaxes chest, FACILITATES QI FLOW, activates the channel, regulates Qi and Blood

Heart 7—Spirit Gate
Location—On the transverse crease of the wrist in a depression on the radial side of the tendon of the Flexor Carpi Ulnaris Muscle
Functions—CALMS SPIRIT AND STRENGTHENS BRAIN, regulates and tonifies the Heart, clears heat, fire, deficiency heat, and heat in the blood.

Small Intestine (SI) 3—Back Stream
location— Lateral to the head of the 5th Metacarpal Bone at the top of the transverse crease formed by a clenched fist
Functions—OPENS THE GOVERNING VESSEL, calms the Spirit, activates the channel and alleviates pain, releases exterior conditions, drains pathogenic influences from Heart, benefits sensory organs, clears fire and heat

Urinary Bladder (UB) 23—Kidneys Hollow
Location—1.5 Body Units lateral to the spinous process of the second Lumbar Vertebrae.
Functions—TONIFIES KIDNEYS, SOURCE QI, ESSENCE AND QI. Nourishes Kidney Yin; regulates the water passages and benefits urination; benefits eyes and ears; strengthens brain, low back, and knees; benefits uterus.

UB 62—Extending Vessel
Location—In a depression directly below the external malleolus
Functions—OPENS AND REGULATES YANG CHIAO MAI, calms Spirit, relaxes muscle channels, activates the channels and relieves pain, clears heat and fire, expels external wind, pacifies internal wind.

Kidney (K) 1—Gushing Spring
Location—On the sole of the foot one third of the distance between the base of the 2nd toe and the heel.
Functions—CONNECTS BODY WITH EARTH AND ABSORBS YIN FROM THE EARTH, tonifies Kidney and Essence, calms Spirit, restores Yang, revives consciousness, clears fire and heat.

K6—Shining Sea
Location—one Body Inch below the medial malleolus
Functions—REGULATES YIN CHIAO MAI, nourishes Kidneys, clears deficiency fire, calms Spirit, regulates the Lower Heater, benefits throat

Pericardium (P) 6—Inner Gate
Location—Two Body Inches above the midpoint of the transverse crease of the wrist between the tendons..
Functions—OPENS THE YIN WEI MAI; regulates and tonifies the Heart, harmonizes the Stomach, eliminates phlegm, clears Heart fire, calms Spirit, suppresses pain, facilitates Qi flow.

P 7—Great Mound
Location—On the transverse wrist crease at the midpoint between tendons of Palmaris Longus and Flexor Carpi Radialis.
Functions—CALMS THE SPIRIT AND CLEARS THE BRAIN, clears Heart fire, unbinds chest, cools heat in the blood, and regulates the Stomach.

P8—Palace of Toil
Location—Between the 2nd and 3rd Metacarpal Bone where tip of middle finger touches the palm when the fingers are held in a half fist.
Functions—MAJOR POINT ON UPPER EXTREMITY TO EMIT AND ABSORB QI, clears heat from the Pericardium and Heart, regulates Heart, calms the Spirit, clears heat from the middle heater, cools heat in the blood, revives consciousness and clears the brain, harmonizes the Stomach.

P 9—Middle Rushing
Location—Center of the tip of the middle finger
Functions—REGULATES THE HEART. Clears Heart fire and heat, benefits the tongue, restores collapsed Yang, restores consciousness

Triple Burner (TB) 4—Yang Pool
Location—In a depression on the back of the hand lateral to the tendon of the Extensor Digitorum Muscle at the level of the wrist joint.
Functions—SOURCE POINT OF THE TRIPLE HEATER, clears heat, relaxes the sinews.

TB 5—Outer Pass
Location—Two Body Inches above TB4 in a depression between the Radius and Ulna

Functions—OPENS YANG WEI MAI, activates the channel, relieves pain, clears heat, tonifies Defensive Qi, relieves exterior conditions

TB 10—Heavens Well
Location—In a depression one Body Inch above the Olecranon
Functions—DESCENDS REBELLIOUS QI DOWNWARDS, expands and relaxes the chest, transforms phlegm, calms the Spirit, clears the brain, clears heat from the channel, activates the channel and relieves pain.

Gall Bladder (GB) 21—Shoulder Well
Location—On the highest point of the shoulder between GV 14 and the Acromion
Functions—DIRECTS QI DOWNWARDS, spreads Liver Qi. clears heat, softens hard masses, expedites labor

GB26—Girdle Vessel
Location—Level with the navel below the free end of the 11th rib
Functions—REGULATES THE GIRDLE VESSEL, transforms damp heat.

GB41—Foot Governor of Tears
Location—In a depression in front of the junction of the 4th and 5th Metacarpal Bones
Functions—CLEARS AND REGULATES THE GIRDLE CHANNEL, spreads Liver and Gall Bladder Qi, clears head and brightens the eyes, transforms phlegm.

Conception Vessel (CV) 1—Meeting of Yin
Location—At the Perineum midway between the anus and sexual organ
Functions—CALMS SPIRIT AND SECURES ESSENCE, clears brain, revives consciousness, tonifies and regulates Qi, clears heat

CV 6—Sea of Qi
Location—One and a half Body Units directly below the umbilicus
Functions—TONIFIES SOURCE QU, KIDNEYS, AND QI; ENRICHES YIN; HARMONIZES AND TONIFIES BLOOD; regulates the Conception Vessel and menstruation; regulates the Lower Heater and water passageways, resolves dampness, damp heat, and damp cold; cools heat in blood, clears deficiency heat, ACTIVATES AND MOBILIZES PRENATAL QI.

CV17—Chest Center—Upper Sea of Qi
Location—In a depression on the Sternum midway between the nipples
Functions—MEETING POINT OF QI, TONIFIES ANCESTRAL QI; regulates the Lungs and Upper Heater, transforms phlegm, regulates and tonifies Qi; unbinds chest; directs rebellious Qi downwards; facilitates lactation.

Governing Vessel (GV) 4—Ming Men—Gate of Life
Location—On the posterior midline in a depression below the spinous process of the second Lumbar Vertebrae.
Functions—TONIFIES KIDNEYS, SOURCE QI, AND ESSENCE; regulates water pathways, clears heat, benefits lower back and bones.

GV14—Big Vertebrae
Location—Between the spinous process of the 7th Cervical Vertebrae and the 1st Thoracic Vertebrae
Functions—MEETING PLACE OF ALL YANG MERIDIANS, TONIFIES DEFENSIVE QI, calms the Spirit and clears the brain, expels wind, clears heat, tonifies deficiency.

GV 20—Hundred Meetings
Location—In a depression at the vertex of the head where a line drawn between the tips of both ears crosses the centerline.
Functions—MAJOR LINK BETWEEN MAN AND HEAVEN; clears brain and calms the Spirit; warms and restored Yang; pacifies wind; sedates Liver Yang; secures the lower orifices; nourishes the Sea of Marrow.

Yin Tang—Hall of Impression
Location—Midpoint between eyebrows
Functions—CALMS SPIRIT, dispels wind, benefits nose

POSTSCRIPT

The pictures and instructions above are useful for understanding the energetics of the exercises as explained. In order to do the practice you should get the workout Video Tape which shows the full body movements for each exercise. The Video may be obtained via the Internet by pointing your browser to

http://www.virtualguild.com/elephant

If your group is interested in one of the qualified teachers from the White Elephant Monastery presenting a Buddha Hands Workshop in your area or you wish to attend one of our workshops in Crestone Colorado you can contact us at the above web address or through the address on the ORDER FORM.

The ideas expressed in this work are the result of 32 years of study in Chinese Martial Arts, Medicine, and QiGong. There are other interpretations of Buddha Hand energetics and the other material in this book that are equally valid.

I once asked my teacher what books I should read to deepen my understanding of QiGong. His answer was that I should not bother to read any books because book knowledge had nothing to do with direct experience—which was real.

It is true that all the intellectual knowledge in the world is useless without the direct experience that comes with practice. On the other hand, for some of us, intellectual knowledge is stimulating and can be used to inspire us to do the practice. Some technical information can be transmitted by books, but learning from an accomplished teacher will impart more than mere technical information. The student should progress much faster under the direct guidance of a high level teacher.

My wish for this book is that it will inspire others to PRACTICE and provide a base of information from which to launch further studies for uncovering their personal understanding—which will be unique to each individual.

PRACTICE EVERY DAY

BIBLIOGRAPHY

The Heart of Yoga by T. K. V. Desikachar
Inner Traditions International 1995

CHAKRAS Energy Centers of Transformation by Harish Johari
Destiny Books 1987

Tao and Longevity by Wen Kuan Chu, Ph.D.
Samuel Weiser, Inc. Third Printing 1991

Chinese Qigong Outgoing-Qi therapy by Bi Yongsheng
Shandong Science and Technology Press 1992

Chinese Qigong Therapy
Shandong Science and Technology Press 1985

Qigong Essentials for Health Promotion by Jiao Guorui
China Reconstructs Press Second edition 1990

Energetic Tai Chi Chuan by Larry Johnson
White Elephant Monastery 1989

Magnetic Healing and Meditation by Larry Johnson
White Elephant Monastery 1988

Hatha Yoga Pradipika by Swami Muktibodhananda Saraswati
Sri G. K. kejriwal Bihar School of Yoga

Acupuncture A Comprehensive Text by Shanghai College of Traditional Medicine—translated and edited by John O'Conner and Dan Bensky
Eastland Press 1981

A Manual of Acupuncture by Peter Deadman and Mazin Al-Khafaji
Journal of Chinese Medicine Publications 1998

Ming Men Observing 'Gate of Life' in the Qigong State by Qu Lifang
Journal of Chinese Medicine Number 40 September 1992
Journal of Chinese Medicine Publications

BIBLIOGRAPHY (continued)

Acupuncture Points Images and Functions by Arnie Lade
Eastland Press, Incorporated 1989

ABOUT THE AUTHOR

Larry Johnson has been involved in Energetic Studies for more than 32 of his 55 years .

This work began with training in Chinese Martial Arts and subsequently expanded to include Oriental Medicine, QiGong, and Meditation.

In 1982 he passed the California State Examination for Licensed Acupuncturist and received his Doctor of Oriental Medicine (O.M.D.) degree from the California Acupuncture College in 1983.

In 1978 Larry was given permission to teach Choy Lee Fut Kung Fu by Grandmaster Ming Jew.

Larry's study of Taoist QiGong, Meditation, and Wu Style Tai Chi Chuan under the private tutelage of a Taoist Master from the Hua San Tradition began in 1976 and continues to this day.

ORDER FORM

White Elephant Monastery
P.O. Box 523
San Francisco, CA. 94101

http://www.virtualguild.com/elephant

	ITEM	PRICE	TOTAL
	Energetic Tai Chi Chuan	$9.95	
	Magnetic Healing and Meditation	$12.95	
	18 Buddha Hands Qigong	$24.95	
	18 Buddha Hands Qigong A Medical I Ching Exploration	$24.95	
	18 Buddha Hands QiGong Video	$29.95	
		Subtotal	
	Shipping & Handling	first item $4.00 each additional item $2.00	
		TOTAL	
	Thank You		

Method of Payment

Cash ________ Money Order ________ Check ________

Credit Card MC / VISA

CC# ____ Exp.________

Name:
Adress:
City/State/Zip

Contact **White Elephant Monastery** for
Seminars or On Site Group Consultations

Our awareness of personal suffering
is directly related to our
perceived separation from God